Performance Improvement in Hospitals and Health Systems

Edited by

James R. Langabeer II, FHIMSS, CMA

Associate Professor of Healthcare Management
The University of Texas School of Public Health

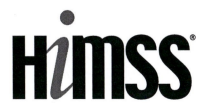

HIMSS Mission

To lead change in the healthcare information and management systems field through knowledge sharing, advocacy, collaboration, innovation, and community affiliations.

ISBN: 978-0-9800697-7-8

For more information about HIMSS, please visit www.himss.org.

"The world hates change, yet it is the only thing that has brought progress."

— Charles Kettering, inventor

About the Editor

James Langabeer II, FHIMSS, CMA, is currently the Chairman of the HIMSS Management Engineering-Process Improvement Committee, an Associate Professor of Management at the University of Texas School of Public Health in Houston, and the Associate Director of the Fleming Center for Healthcare Management. He previously served in leadership capacities for two world-renowned academic medical centers, where he had responsibilities for a variety of functions, including management engineering, budgeting and planning, supply chain operations, financial management, and business analysis. He was also the executive vice president for one of the fastest growing consulting and technology firms in the U.S., where he consulted in over 30 countries globally for the world's leading Fortune 500 firms across healthcare, retail, and manufacturing industries.

Dr. Langabeer holds a bachelor of business administration from the University of Texas at San Antonio, a master of business administration from Baylor University, and a doctorate in leadership and administration from the University of Houston, where his research focused on economic performance and strategic management of large teaching hospitals. Dr. Langabeer is also a Certified Management Accountant and a Fellow of the Healthcare Information and Management Systems Society. He is the author of several books, including *Healthcare Operations Management: A Quantitative Approach to Business and Logistics* (Jones and Bartlett, 2008). He can be contacted at www.Decision-Strategy.com.

About the Contributors

Sandra Blanke, ABD, CISSP, is an Assistant Professor of Information Assurance at the University of Dallas, a Certified Information Systems Security Professional (CISSP), and an enterprise business consultant. Ms. Blanke has an extensive background as a leader and technical director in the telecommunications industry and teaches graduate classes in information security. Ms. Blanke's primary research streams are focused in the areas of contingency planning and disaster recovery, computer abuse in the business environment, Intranet security risks and various other security technologies. In 2008 she will complete her PhD dissertation which is entitled "A Study of the Contributions of Attitude, Computer Security Policy Awareness, and Computer Self Efficacy on the Employees' Computer Abuse Intention in Business Environments."

Kim Brant-Lucich, MBA, PMP, is Director of Process Redesign for St. Joseph Health System in Orange, California. In that role, Ms. Brant-Lucich has developed a comprehensive, reusable methodology for process redesign and change management for system implementation projects. She also works with the various St. Joseph Health System hospitals to align their IT initiatives with business goals and develop their IT strategic road-maps. In addition to her current responsibilities, Ms. Brant-Lucich is also an adjunct professor in the Healthcare Administration Master's Program at California State University at Long Beach. Prior to joining St. Joseph Health System, Ms. Brant-Lucich worked at Kaiser Permanente Health Plan as a senior project manager and at Ernst & Young LLP as a manager in the Healthcare/Managed Care Consulting Practice. She has been involved in numerous projects with managed care organizations and hospital systems, including call center implementations, customer satisfaction survey design and analysis, and customer service visioning. Ms. Brant-Lucich holds an MBA from the University of Southern California Marshall School of Business, and a BA from the University of California at Davis; she is also a certified Project Management Professional. Ms. Brant-Lucich serves as the national Vice Chair of the HIMSS Management Engineering-Process Improvement Committee.

James R. Broyles, BSE, is a PhD candidate in Operations Research at Arizona State University's Industrial Engineering Department. He has work experience in both manufacturing and healthcare engineering. His healthcare experience includes emergency department redesigns, outpatient clinic modeling and facilities layout. Mr. Broyles's dissertation is focused on using probability modeling to approximate patient flows in hospitals.

Rigoberto (Rigo) Delgado, MBA, is a Senior Management Engineer in the Department of Strategic Financial Planning at the University of Texas MD Anderson Cancer Center, Houston, and manages projects related to feasibility studies, performance analysis and strategic planning. Previously, Mr. Delgado worked as a management consultant and as an executive for several organizations. Mr. Delgado holds a BS in Agricultural Economics (honors) from the University of Chihuahua, Mexico, an MBA in Finance from the University of California at Berkeley, and is a doctoral candidate, concentrating on management, in the University of Texas School of Public Health.

Jami DelliFraine, PhD, is an Assistant Professor in the Division of Management, Policy, and Community Health in the School of Public Health at the University of Texas, Houston. Her research focuses on the organization and management of non-profit hospitals, including safety-net hospitals and rural hospitals. She has published her research in journals such as *Health Care Management Review, Hospital Topics, Health Marketing Quarterly* and *Journal of Health Care Finance.* Some of her research is currently supported by the Center for Rural Pennsylvania and the National Institute of Mental Health. She teaches Quality Management, Management of Health Services Organizations, and Understanding Organizational Behavior in Health Services Organizations. She graduated from Virginia Commonwealth University in 2004 with a PhD in Health Services Organization and Research.

John Hansmann, MSIE, CPHIMS, FHIMSS, DSHS, is the Urban South Region Manager of Management Engineering for Intermountain Healthcare, Salt Lake City. He has more than 20 years of healthcare experience in operations, strategy and IT analysis. His current focus is facilitating the development of standardized nursing care models and staffing practices, optimizing patient throughput and leading the workflow analysis supporting Intermountain's development of a state-of-the-art clinical information system in partnership with GE Healthcare. Mr. Hansmann is a Fellow of HIMSS and is the board liaison to both the Advocacy and Public Policy Steering Committee and the CPHIMS Technical Committee. Mr. Hansmann has been an active member of HIMSS, serving on numerous committees such as CPHIMS committee (chair), Health Leadership Alliance Expert Panel, Annual Conference Education Committee and elected member of the Nominating Committee. He has been an annual conference paper reviewer/coach and presenter numerous times. Mr. Hansmann was the author of two chapters in the *HIMSS Guidebook Series: Management Engineering.* In 2002, he received the prestigious HIMSS Leadership Award. Mr. Hansmann is also a senior member of the Institute of Industrial Engineers (IIE), and Diplomate within the Society for Health Systems (DSHS), a society within IIE. He has served in many different roles in IIE and SHS, culminating with being the national President for SHS in 1999/2000. Mr. Hansmann received his BSIE and MSIE from North Dakota State University.

Margaret J. Holm, MHSA, FACHE, is a healthcare executive in Houston. Previously, she was an executive director at MD Anderson Cancer Center, a position in which she taught clinical quality and safety improvement methods with an evidence-based approach and developed organizational infrastructures to facilitate change in care delivery. Throughout her career, Ms. Holm has improved organizational performance by developing teams to focus on patient care delivery processes and utilize data as a tool for effective decision-making. As CEO of a community hospital, Ms. Holm was responsible for developing the hospital strategy with the governing body and medical leadership, managing physician office practices, coordinating health plans, ensuring regulatory and standard compliance, improving quality of care and lowering operational costs. As a nursing faculty member, she taught introductory and management skills to nursing students. As a nurse providing direct care, she worked in critical care. She has served as a member of an advisory council for The Joint Commission, Governing Council for the American Hospital Association, Board of Directors for Utah Healthcare Association and Adjunct Faculty for Weber State University. She is a fellow in the American College of Healthcare Executives. Ms. Holm received her graduate degree in Health Services Administration from Ohio University and her BSN from the University of Utah.

Roger Kropf, PhD, is a Professor in the Health Policy and Management Program at New York University's Robert F. Wagner Graduate School of Public Service. Dr. Kropf is the author of several books on the application of information systems to healthcare management. *Strategic Analysis for Hospital Management* was written with James Greenberg, PhD, and published by Aspen Systems in 1984. *Service Excellence in Healthcare through the Use of Computers* was published by the American College of Healthcare Executives in 1990. His most recent book, *Making Information Technology Work: Maximizing the Benefits for Healthcare Organizations,* was co-written with Guy Scalzi and published by AHA Press in 2007. He teaches graduate and executive education courses on information technology. More information on his work can be found at his Web site, www.nyu.edu/classes/kropf.

Leon J. Leach, MBA, MA, is an Executive Vice President at the University of Texas MD Anderson Cancer Center. His responsibilities include executive leadership for the business, administrative and support departments including finance, business development, marketing, human resources, facilities management, information services, and technology development and commercialization. In addition, he also serves as the Chairman of the Board of Directors of MD Anderson Services Corporation, an Anderson-controlled entity that facilitates and invests in early-stage start-up companies based on institutionally invented technologies. Prior to this, Mr. Leach was executive vice president and chief financial officer at Cornerstone Physicians Corporation in Irvine, California, and was the senior vice president for operations and chief financial officer with CareAmerica Health Plans Inc., a southern California-based $600 million health maintenance organization. Prior to joining CareAmerica, Mr. Leach served as senior vice president and chief financial officer of Candle SubAcute Services Inc., also in southern California. Candle was the largest privately held manager of subacute healthcare facilities in California prior to its purchase by Vencor Hospitals, Inc. Mr. Leach spent 25 years in various leadership positions at the Prudential Insurance Company of America, serving as senior vice president of the Prudential Healthcare Plan (PruCare), and subsequently as senior vice president and chief financial officer of the Prudential Real Estate Affiliates. He was instrumental in the establishment and start-up operations of 18 health maintenance organizations throughout the southeast and eastern U.S. while with Prudential. Mr. Leach holds a master's degree from Southwestern Baptist Theological Seminary, an MBA from Widener University, and a bachelor's degree from Rutgers University.

Elizabeth McGrady, PhD, FACHE, is an Assistant Professor and the Academic Program Director for the Health Services Management MBA program at the University of Dallas. She has worked in the healthcare field for more than 30 years as a clinician, executive, educator and consultant. She received her PhD in community health from the University of Tennessee and has a Master's of Healthcare Administration from Tulane University, and a Master's of Education and Bachelor's of Science in Medical Technology from the University of Florida. In addition to teaching healthcare management courses, Dr. McGrady provides strategic, business and marketing planning consulting services. She is a Fellow of the American College of Healthcare Executives.

Cynthia McKinney, MBA, FHIMSS, is a Healthcare Consultant in the Strategic and Change–Clinical Transformation/Health Analytics practice at IBM. She has more than 24 years of experience in healthcare and IT. She is skilled in health analytics, management engineering and project management. She has an in-depth background in value realization and process optimization for IT and facility initiatives. Ms. McKinney has excellent financial management skills consisting of analysis and interpretation. She is effective in preparing and facilitating presentations, design sessions, and training. She also has an extensive background in decision support systems. Ms. McKinney is an active participant in the healthcare IT industry, having recently been recognized in 2007 with the SIG Leadership Award from HIMSS, two Spirit of HIMSS Awards in 2006, and the HIMSS 2004 Board of Directors Award. A HIMSS Fellow since 1998, Ms. McKinney has served on the HIMSS Board of Directors, as chair of the Management Engineering-Process Improvement Task Force and as the founding member/president of the Heart of America Chapter of HIMSS.

Osama Mikhail, PhD, serves as Senior Vice President, Strategic Planning at the University of Texas, Health Science Center-Houston. He is also a Professor of Management and Policy Sciences at the University of Texas, School of Public Health. At the school, Dr. Mikhail teaches courses in healthcare finance, planning and management, and advises students in both the masters and doctoral programs. Previously, Dr. Mikhail served in a number of capacities at St. Luke's Episcopal Health System in Houston, including chief planning and chief strategic officer and senior vice president, planning, development and academic affairs. Dr. Mikhail received a BS in math and physics from the American University of Beirut in Lebanon, an MBA in finance from the University of Pennsylvania's Wharton School, and an MS in industrial administration and PhD in systems sciences from the Graduate School of Industrial Administration at Carnegie-Mellon University in Pittsburgh.

Kevin T. Roche, MSIE, PhD, recently completed his doctorate in Industrial Engineering from Arizona State University's Ira A. Fulton School of Engineering. He received his bachelor's and master's degrees from ASU. His dissertation is titled "Whole Hospital

Analytical Modeling and Control." Along with Dr. Jeffery Cochran, he has been working on applying industrial engineering and operations research tools and thinking to solve problems in many aspects of the healthcare system.

Guy Scalzi, MBA, is a Principal Consultant with Aspen Advisors LLC, where he works with a number of healthcare provider organizations. Previously he was executive vice president of Veloz Global, a software and services company based in Mt. View, California, with development and support offices in India. He has also held the position of managing director of outsourcing services at First Consulting Group, CIO at New York Presbyterian Healthcare in New York City and president of DataEase International, a Connecticut-based software company. He spent 14 years as a hospital administrator in New York City before moving into information systems. He is an adjunct assistant professor at New York University's Robert F. Wagner Graduate School of Public Service, where he teaches courses on information management in healthcare. He is the coauthor (with Roger Kropf) of *Making Information Technology Work: Maximizing the Benefits for Healthcare Organizations* (Health Forum/AHA Press, 2007). He received his MBA in finance from Manhattan College.

Contents

Preface

The need for change and improvement in healthcare has never been greater. As medical costs continue to escalate at rates nearly triple those in other industries, the outcomes, quality and cost-effectiveness of healthcare processes become center stage for every hospital or healthcare system. In the United States, healthcare expenditures represent more than $2 trillion annually, which is equal to four times the national defense budget, or approximately $7,500 per person. It is well recognized that a big part of this expense is purely waste—waste in terms of duplication of effort, over-utilization of resources, and inefficient administration and clinical processes. Although shifts in federal government and macro-level policy may create change in the long term, if change is to occur in the near term, it must come from within organizations. Who do these organizations— hospitals, clinics and systems—look to for answers in promoting change internally?

A growing number of successful systems are recruiting and developing specialized professionals who can lead and facilitate internal change. That is the role of management engineers (MEs) and performance improvement (PI) professionals. As process and system experts, these professionals must begin to play a broader role in redefining healthcare in the U.S. by constructing cost-effective healthcare within our hospitals and health systems. You might ask: What is the role and purpose of an ME or a performance analyst, and why should healthcare organizations invest in them? Just as clinics and hospitals need physicians and nurses, as technology becomes more integrated and central to patient care, IT professionals will become as essential. However, only a small minority fully understands and appreciates the potential of professionals dedicated to improving, on a daily basis, the performance of management systems, workflow and outcomes, certainly a valuable and substantial contribution.

Industrial engineering techniques have been applied to healthcare since the early 1900s. While industrial engineers such as Frank and Lillian Gilbreth focused on process efficiency, others such as Frederick Taylor worked on improving productivity using time and motion studies. Together, these early pioneers demonstrated to surgeons and providers that the healthcare industry could benefit from process improvement much the same as manufacturing industries had. For healthcare, this meant redesigning the clinician's workflow to increase outputs in the operating room. The field was significantly advanced by Harold Smalley, one of the founding fathers of the Healthcare Management Systems Society—which later became the Healthcare Information and Management Systems Society (HIMSS). Since that time, we have seen growth in the number of organizations, journals and training opportunities that purport the "science of improvement." However, that growth is insufficient. We need greater penetration of PI specialists using a combination of engineering and organizational development techniques to focus on attacking the obstacles that prevent progress in healthcare.

CONTRIBUTIONS OF ENGINEERS AND ANALYSTS

Through the 12 chapters of this book, we will explore how PI professionals can apply engineering and improvement techniques to change processes. As many PI consultants are engineers, we will start with a basic definition: **Management Engineering** in the healthcare arena can be defined as the application of engineering principles to healthcare processes. It can also be defined as a discipline focused on designing optimal management and information systems and processes, using tools from engineering, mathematics and social sciences. More specifically, ME involves analyzing processes and decisions using a framework that:

- Ensures decisions are analytical and data-driven. MEs tend to express variables and activities in quantitative terms, using actual data obtained from information systems or calculated from observations.
- Embodies an engineering approach, in which science is applied to decision making. This engineering approach completely supports the current trend toward evidence-based medicine, which permits data to drive decision making, rather than it being driven by assumptions and intuitions.
- Focuses on a systems perspective. This not only includes information systems but also management systems, or interconnecting processes and procedures.
- Incorporates cost-effectiveness, or the relationships between incremental value produced from a process and its associated costs. Since most gains in performance are derived only from commitment to additional expenses, such as investing in new technology or equipment, MEs can play a valuable role in identifying useful practices that have high cost-effectiveness, thereby ensuring that resources are optimally applied.

These functions are shown in Figure 1.

Whereas industrial engineers from the past can be classified best as tacticians or technicians, today's analysts are best described as change agents. As internal consultants who help executives better manage projects and who serve as leaders of key IT and capital projects, they use collaboration and facilitation skills to guide team efforts and understand performance drivers and technology better than anyone in the organization to help make changes stick. As PI has become an issue for the boardroom, now is the time for engineers and analysts to expand their toolkits and take a visible, leadership role in organizational change.

The breadth and scope of PI professionals is growing. A small sample of the projects that MEs or performance analysts help lead is shown in Table 1.

ABOUT THIS BOOK

I should make a few points for clarification here. First, anytime we use the term *performance improvement* (or *PI*) professional, we are primarily talking about internal consultants who use a combination of methods to change systems and processes. Some organizations call these consultants *management engineers* or *industrial engineers,* and many are known by other names—operations analyst, process consultant, project manager, "black belt," Six Sigma consultant, business process analyst, management analyst and quality manager—just to name a few. Small differences aside, all of these are key staff positions through which professionals help lead change and improve

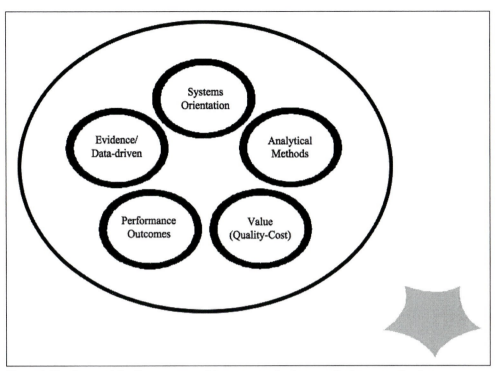

Figure 1: The Focus of the Contemporary Management Engineer or Performance Analyst

Table 1: Typical Performance Improvement Projects

Implementation of systems and technology	New facility construction projects
Development of business plans	Process workflow redesign
Performance benchmarking	Productivity and staffing management
Supply chain reengineering	Simulation modeling of clinics and units
Cataloging and deploying "evidence" to improve medical quality	Data mining for decision making

performance. You will notice that we will use these terms interchangeably in this book, but truthfully, every administrator and executive who devotes his or her time to making things better and not just maintaining the status quo is a PI professional.

Another point of clarification is that as the field of PI is rapidly expanding, it is difficult (or impossible) to find any one expert who understands the theory and practice of all the methods used in advanced health systems. Understanding this prompted me to turn to a number of colleagues and recognized experts, individuals with extensive practical or scholarly knowledge in this area. These experts will share their methods, results and best practices. Each of these authors brings his or her unique experience and perspective, as well as a passion for the topic. As a result, the book is a comprehensive analysis in this field.

A third clarification is to note that this book is not intended to be theoretical in nature. Rather, my hope is that readers find it to be applicable, practical and actionable. Healthcare organizations have a long way to go to master their process workflows, information and management systems and overall performance. It is my expectation that this book will significantly advance the discussion by providing valuable insights into what practitioners are doing to improve and maintain their environments.

With that said, this book is specifically written for those in health systems who are charged with avoiding the status quo and the comfort zone in delivering results. Executives, administrators, managers, analysts, physicians, nurses and pharmacists all will benefit from a better understanding of process and performance improvement. This is meant as a timely and relevant book as hospitals, clinics and systems begin or continue their improvement journeys. I hope the information therein contributes to an improved outcome.

Acknowledgments

With deep gratitude, I acknowledge the outstanding contributions of those who helped to create this book. More than a dozen industry leaders and academics, each with an inestimable background in his or her area of expertise, offer refreshing perspectives on performance improvement. Without them, the book would not have been as rich in information and diverse in experience.

I also thank Fran Perveiler, vice president of communications, and JoAnn Klinedinst, vice president of education, both at HIMSS. Their recognition of the value of management engineering and performance improvement is reflected in the help they provided in moving this book from concept to reality. I appreciate the leadership HIMSS commands in this topical area.

I also appreciate the support of Rhonda Ruiz, CPA, for her detailed reviews and critiques of manuscripts. In addition, I would not be nearly as productive without the conducive environment created by my students and colleagues at the University of Texas Health Science Center at Houston. Finally, the guidance provided by Dave Worthington, PhD, a world-renowned operations research expert at Lancaster University Management School, is also greatly appreciated.

Finally, I am grateful to have a wife who is very supportive of my interest in improving the healthcare system. I dedicate this book to her—Denise Langabeer.

SECTION I

HEALTHCARE PERFORMANCE

As this book is about engineering positive changes or improvements in the healthcare system, we need to begin with a thorough definition of performance as it relates to health systems. The term *performance* means different things to different people, depending on perspective and setting. In the retail industry, customers might consider performance to be the quality of the product they are buying, whereas retail executives might view it as return on assets or same-store year-over-year sales growth. In healthcare, performance is a broad and complicated topic. To a provider, performance often suggests technical quality measures, while a board of trustees might consider performance in financial terms. It is very multidimensional term, as we describe in this book.

Section I of this book provides the reader with the basics of performance—what it is, and why employees, managers, physicians, nurses, and healthcare organizations must focus on it. Most people think they understand "good" performance, but hospitals and health systems are atypical organizations; what defines performance and success in hospitals and health systems is significantly different than that of other industries. Likewise, whereas many physicians and administrators define performance in narrow, abstract terms, the performance improvement (PI) professional seeks to define the term with far greater precision and breadth. Unless analysts have a comprehensive understanding of all the different performance outcomes, it is very difficult to achieve any gains or realize any benefits.

To begin to understand different perspectives, Chapter 1 helps to define executives' perception of performance and their expectations from PI professionals. A strategic perspective is offered from Leon Leach, a senior executive at MD Anderson Cancer Center, Houston, one of the most respected institutions in the world. He discusses the role that performance analysts should play and defines the outcomes senior leadership expects and desires from performance improvement efforts. This chapter describes the technical gap that exists between the profession and its executives and how that gap has slowed adoption rates of PI methods. This gap is all too often caused by our overuse of technical jargon, buzzwords, and models that are not understood by those executives to whom we have presented our ideas. Without a clear understanding, executives are likely to ignore or minimize the potential contribution of process improvement initiatives.

Chapter 1 creates the foundation for PI as a strategic contribution to the organization, and provides tips on how to better align process improvement with strategic goals.

In Chapter 2, Osama Mikhail, Jami DelliFraine, and I define organizational performance from the healthcare perspective. We discuss the performance-strategy relationship, describe performance targets and define a framework. Without a comprehensive perspective on performance, it is impossible to understand what to improve, let alone set standards, goals and plans for the future. Using a strategic approach, projects should first focus on desired performance impacts, then map out plans and performance targets. A performance framework is offered for better categorizing performance variables.

Chapter 3 defines a "benefit realization" framework for recognizing benefits in healthcare process and technology projects. *Benefits* are those quantitative gains in performance accrued to a process as a result of focused effort from a well-coordinated project. Cindy McKinney, one of the most recognized management engineers in healthcare and a senior managing consultant with IBM Consulting in Kansas City, Missouri, describes her time-tested approach to benefit realization.

CHAPTER 1

The Executive Perspective on Performance Improvement

Leon J. Leach

"Nothing is an obstacle unless you say it is."
— Wally Amos, Famous Amos Cookies

INTRODUCTION

Those involved in the delivery of healthcare are in for rough sailing over the next several years. Most observers believe our current healthcare system is broken. There is plenty of blame to go around, with fingers pointed at providers, third-party payers, the uninsured, consumers, the over-utilizers, Big Pharma, baby boomers (for aging), the U.S. Congress, U.S. presidents (past and current), and many more. Everyone shares responsibility for the current situation.

Setting blame aside, prominent leaders across all industries agree that our healthcare system is broken or, at the least, is not providing satisfactory value for the resources consumed. California Governor Arnold Schwarzenegger has flatly declared that his state's "healthcare system is broken."[1] His plan to fix the California healthcare system died in the legislative process. Members of our nation's largest union, the AFL-CIO, collectively believe that the entire U.S. healthcare system is broken,[2] with others from very divergent walks of life agreeing, such as Newt Gingrich, who has presented his own plan to transform healthcare.[3] Michael Moore, famous for his movie *Sicko*,[4] offers three easy steps to fix the healthcare problem: (1) provide to everyone free care for life; (2) abolish health insurance companies; and (3) regulate pharmaceutical companies as utilities. And, of course, in an election year every presidential candidate has his or her plan to fix the system. Finally, the supposed beneficiary of the system, the American consumer, is also dissatisfied and thinks the system is broken.[5] Porter and Teisberg, in their research on competition for value in healthcare, sum up the national situation quite well:

> No one is happy with the current system—not patients, who worry about the cost of insurance and the quality of care; not employers, who face escalating premiums and unhappy employees; not physicians

and other providers, whose incomes have been squeezed, professional judgments overridden, and workdays overwhelmed with bureaucracy and paperwork; not health plans, which are routinely vilified; not suppliers of drugs and medical devices, which have introduced many life-saving or life enhancing therapies but get blamed for driving up costs; and not governments, whose budgets are spinning out of control.[6]

The conclusion is obvious: unless healthcare leaders transform the system; that is, provide more value for the resources consumed, other catalysts will drive the change. These could include congressional action that would, essentially, nationalize healthcare. Alternatively, a catalyst could be third-party payers, including the government, eroding reimbursements to levels at which the healthcare system is subsequently changed, for better or worse. Or, a catalyst might be as simple as the competitor down the street actually figuring out how to deliver more value from fewer resources, forcing organizations to change or go out of business.

THE CASE FOR VALUE

In other fields, huge gains have been made by better integrating the activities required to serve customers. Healthcare, according to Porter and Teisberg, is well overdue for such a transformation. They cite the University of Texas MD Anderson Cancer Center, Houston, as one example of success, using such innovation. MD Anderson has integrated all the relevant medical specialties for patient care into centers, according to the type of cancer for which a patient is being treated, a change about which the authors remark: "Patient value is enhanced by organizing practice around medical conditions in tailored facilities, rather than shuttling the patient among numerous offices and departments. These are not focused factories, but sets of facilities or areas within larger facilities that integrate the care cycle."[7]

Simply reorganizing into a more patient-centric environment will not, in and of itself, drive value; more sophisticated tools are needed. Healthcare in the future is all about delivering value, not simply reducing costs, but changing the nature of the relationship between inputs and outputs to increase value to consumers. Better health per dollar spent is the goal, according to most stakeholders, thereby decreeing healthcare leaders to employ better tools to achieve this value proposition. At MD Anderson, we rely heavily on performance improvement (PI) tools to make this happen.

PI is approaching "motherhood and apple pie" in terms of its perceived virtue. It is not simply a matter of working harder; rather, it is a matter of, to use the old adage, "working smarter." The value of engaging in continuous performance improvement is obvious; financial performance, degrees of quality and customer satisfaction can all be generally enhanced. In the world of healthcare, quality and patient satisfaction are the dominant missions of systems and somewhat overshadow the issue of financial performance as key organizational goals, although all are important. In short, there are overwhelmingly positive reasons to engage in a serious continuous performance effort in your organization. So, let us look at the flip side of the coin: reasons why PI is sometimes resisted.

EXECUTIVE RESISTANCE TO PERFORMANCE IMPROVEMENT

Executives often resist programs and processes they do not understand, which is why it is essential to make PI relevant to the organization by avoiding the following common pitfalls:

Make PI Relevant

Some view performance improvement as a recycling of Frederick Winslow Taylor's Scientific Management concept,[8] which dates back to the 1880s. They are correct; PI does have many of its roots in Taylor's classic *Principles of Scientific Management*, written in 1911, and his studies with Bethlehem Steel Works in the 1880s. Subsequent researchers built on these theories and advanced Taylor's work while adding concepts of their own. Although the traditional stopwatch employed in their infamous time and motion studies of a century ago were breakthroughs of the day, today's tools are much more sophisticated and are fresh, new and particularly relevant to healthcare. Today's continuous PI concepts are not your grandfather's time and motion studies.

Don't Let Language Be a Barrier

New, sophisticated concepts that have developed in the field lead to the next challenge—the language used by continuous PI experts. What, specifically, is meant by data mining, queuing, simulation modeling, Six Sigma, PDCA (Plan-Do-Check-Act, which is explained later), Delphi technique, focused brainstorming, how-how tree diagram, mindmapping, process decision contingency chart, 5 whys and 1 how, Pareto diagram, affinity diagram, and, my personal favorite, the why-why tree diagram? The specialized expressions (read "gobbledygook") generally associated with continuous PI are often confusing or intimidating to executives at best and a rare form of torture at worst. Is this ever-expanding vernacular really necessary? Can we not simplify the language to help make the exchange of concepts a little easier?

Performance improvement language can be frustrating and may leave an impression with the chief executive officer (perhaps even more so with the chief financial officer) that continuous PI is somehow related to that Shakespearean comedy, *Much Ado About Nothing*. Executives need to understand that all professions have a unique language and do their best to embrace it to the point of becoming conversant in the field. For their part, PI analysts must avoid allowing language to become a barrier. To help the reader to also avoid this obstacle and become well versed in this language, a glossary of key terms is included in this book.

Ensure That PI Adds Value

Many CFOs and CEOs might believe that PI programs incur significant costs, in terms of labor, consultants, interdisciplinary teams, software, training and supplies. To avoid this perception, the focus of PI needs to be fixed on value delivered, not on costs. Value is expressed as the incremental change in quality or outcomes derived from specific investment. Managing PI projects appropriately requires that upfront analysis be conducted prior to accepting projects, to ensure that value creation can occur. Managing and maintaining projects using this same philosophy also ensure that results are worth the effort. Done right, using good tools focused on benefit realization, PI will lead to better organizational outcomes. In the subsequent chapters, we will discuss the use of value-added project management tools to ensure that PI adds value.

THE BENEFITS OF PERFORMANCE IMPROVEMENT

Dismissing the time-honored objections referred to earlier, let's get to the point of why we need PI—it works. In the broadest sense, continuous PI is about making life better through improved quality. In the healthcare world, specifically, PI may be the tool that keeps healthcare professionals in charge of the healthcare system in the U.S.

Performance improvement is often brought on board when it is recognized that there is a need to reduce operating expenses. Its implementation often accomplishes that but also leads to a better way of doing things, not only by saving money but also through an improved quality of life. Let's take an example from outside the healthcare industry. Tolko Industries LTD, a 52-year-old Canadian company (with corporate headquarters in Vernon, BC) manufactures specialty forest products such as wood beams and panels. Tolko is a substantial company employing more than 4,500 people with $1.9 billion in annual sales revenue.[9] Faced with increasing natural gas costs in 2004, Tolko management embarked on a revolutionary strategy to convert operations to a bioreactor producing clean-burning synthetic natural gas from wood bark. Bark sales had formerly produced only modest revenue for Tolko but using bark as an alternative fuel, management realized $1.5 million in energy savings, which established Tolko as the sole low-cost producer of specialty forest products.[10]

An improved bottom line was not the only benefit. Tolko received the Canadian Industry Program for Energy Conservation Leadership Award for reducing greenhouse gas emissions. Michael Towers, Manager, Tolko Energy Supply and Systems, recalls that "increasing our competitive advantage by reducing our operating costs was a primary goal for Tolko." But, "to do it in a way that also dramatically reduced our greenhouse gas emissions really made it a win-win solution for us."[11] Not only did Tolko derive financial benefits from PI, but achieved better health through a cleaner environment as a second happy outcome. This same combination—a better bottom line and higher quality for patients—is often the result of continuous PI in healthcare.

Rather than being mutually exclusive, patient safety, more efficient operations, and patient and employee satisfaction go hand-in-hand with enhanced operating margins. Margins are essential to any healthcare entity or to any going concern for that matter. Sister Irene Kraus of the Daughters of Charity is credited with coining the phrase; "no margin, no mission."

A STUDY OF PERFORMANCE IMPROVEMENT AT MD ANDERSON

One could argue that patient benefits, starting with safety, are the "raison d'être" for continuous PI in the healthcare field. PI efforts at my institution, the University of Texas MD Anderson Cancer Center in Houston, date at least back to the late 1990s. The success of this effort can be told one story at a time, or by reviewing higher level performance metrics. Let's quickly do a little of both but, first, some background on the plan itself.

MD Anderson's Aim for Excellence Performance Improvement Plan is detailed in an 11-page document.[12] The plan is aligned with the institution's mission, vision and values and is directed by the Institutional Quality Council, which is co-chaired by the executive vice president and physician-in-chief and the vice president for performance improvement and chief quality officer. The Quality Council includes approximately two dozen members from all areas of the institution and also includes several rotational members selected each year based on annual strategic plan initiatives. The Quality Council interrelates across the institution and is strongly supported by executive leadership in all areas. Among its responsibilities, the Quality Council reviews and prioritizes improvement projects using the following criteria regarding the project's:

- Alignment with strategic vision and goals
- Relation to patient safety
- Concern with high volume, high risk, high cost and/or problem-prone areas
- Relation to customer satisfaction
- Relation to financial goals (cost reduction and/or revenue generation)

The methodology followed is the Plan-Do-Check-Act (PDCA) process made popular by Deming[13] in his work on process control. A report is issued for each project, including an estimate of savings and value enhancement. Projects are staffed either with teams chartered by the Quality Council to address major cross-functional programs or by registered teams used for less complex challenges. Staffing for the projects can come from the involved areas and the Office of the Vice President for Performance Improvement and the chief quality officer.

To have more people trained and involved in these areas, MD Anderson started a Transformation Specialist Program in 2003, selecting high-potential employees in patient service areas to spend one year in an educational and experiential residency within the Office of Performance Improvement. On completion of the program, the individual returns to his or her patient service area as an in-house "performance improvement specialist." This effort to train and embed experts within the line areas further strengthens a commitment to performance improvement.[14]

Two brief examples of the achieved success that was driven by commitment to PI include the Healthcare Alliance Safety Partnership (HASP) and the Multidisciplinary Antimicrobial Stewardship Team (MAST). HASP is a joint project between MD Anderson and the State of Texas Board of Nursing to evaluate possible changes in the relationship between the regulatory agency and the practice environment. Patterned after the Aviation Safety Action Program, in which near-misses are self-reported and jointly analyzed for possible systemic changes by the regulatory body and the industry, the HASP pilot program has been deemed successful by the Texas Board of Nursing, and they are expanding the program to other hospitals. During the first year of the pilot, an incident involving the inadvertent administration of a feeding tube into an intravenous line was analyzed. The result is a change in the universality of the connectors to prevent feeding tubes from being inadvertently connected to intravenous lines.[15]

MAST arose from an antibiotic stewardship project conducted in MD Anderson's Clinical Safety and Effectiveness course. A multidisciplinary project team, using PI tools, was able to improve by more than 45% the appropriate usage of antimicrobial drugs in the intensive care unit. As a result, lengths of stay, mortality rates and readmission rates decreased. The outcomes will result in a substantial expense savings over time.[16]

The two efforts, HASP and MAST, are specific examples of PI changing the environment for the better at MD Anderson. Higher level performance metrics, such as the operating margin, patient satisfaction and patient safety, have significantly improved since MD Anderson embraced PI in the late 1990s. Further, MD Anderson has been consistently named as one of the top cancer centers in the nation by *U.S. News and World Report*. Performance improvement may be coincidental or it may be causal; we do not know for sure. But, we are not going to suspend our PI efforts to ascertain whether a causal relationship does, in fact, exist.

SUMMARY

One way or another, U.S. healthcare will be transformed. The goal must now be a focus on better health per dollar spent. The transformation either will be lead by healthcare organizations striving to improve their value propositions or it will be forced by outside pressures. Changes forced from outside the industry may be more draconian and may, fundamentally, miss the point. Price and cost, which will likely be the focus of forced change, are not the same as value. Lower cost does not necessarily increase value. Social goodwill is better served by the healthcare industry leading the effort to generate better health per dollar spent. Performance improvement is one of the primary tools available to the healthcare industry to accomplish this step.

References

1. State of California. Office of the Governor. *Fixing Our Broken Healthcare System*. 2007. Available at: www.fixourhealthcare.ca.gov. Accessed March 1, 2008.
2. Michaels S. Broken Healthcare System Costs Employers and Employees. *AFL-CIO Now Blog News*. 2008. Available at: http://blog.aflcio.org/2008/02/15/broken-health-care-system-costs-employers-and-employees/.
3. Gingrich N. *Saving Lives and Saving Money: Transforming Health and Healthcare*. Washington, DC: Alexis de Tocqueville Institution; 2003.
4. Moore M. Michael Moore's Healthcare Proposal. Available at: http://www.michaelmoore.com/sicko/health-care-proposal. Accessed February 10, 2008.
5. Zwillich T. U.S. Trails Others in Healthcare Satisfaction. FoxNews.com. October 29, 2004.
6. Porter M, Teisberg EO. *Redefining Healthcare: Creating Value Based Competition on Results*. Boston: Harvard Business School Press; 2006.
7. Porter M, Teisberg EO. How physicians can change the future of healthcare. *JAMA*. 2007; 297:1103-1111.
8. Taylor FW. *The Principles of Scientific Management*. Harper and Brothers Press; 1911.
9. *Tolko Industries Ltd. 2006 Annual Review*. 2006. Available at: www.tolko.com. Accessed February 10, 2008.
10. Tertzakian P. *A Thousand Barrels a Second*. New York: McGraw-Hill; 2007.
11. Canada Newswire. Tolko Industries Receives Energy Conservation Award for Nexterra Gasification System at Heffley Creek Mill. December 20, 2007.
12. The University of Texas MD Anderson Cancer Center. Aim for Excellence Performance Improvement Plan (internal document); 2007.
13. Deming WE. *Out of the Crisis*. MIT Center for Advanced Engineering Study; 1986.
14. The University of Texas MD Anderson Cancer Center. Transformation Specialist Program: Moving Improvement into the Institution (internal document); 2008.
15. Simmons D. *The Healthcare Alliance Safety Partnership: A Translational Research Pilot in Safety*. E-mail to the author. January 24, 2008.
16. Perego C, Adachi J. *Antibiotic Stewardship Initiative in the Intensive Care Unit*. Clinical Safety & Effectiveness (CS&E) Educational Program, Session 4. The University of Texas MD Anderson Cancer Center, Houston. January 12, 2007.

CHAPTER 2

Organizational Performance Management

James Langabeer II, Osama Mikhail and Jami DelliFraine

> *"The thing is, continuity of strategic direction and continuous improvement in how you do things are absolutely consistent with each other. In fact, they're mutually reinforcing."*
> — Michael Porter, Harvard Business School

INTRODUCTION

The concept of improving performance requires that organizations and systems understand their current performance and then develop a vision about future performance levels. In many respects, this visioning process requires that managers approach each project as a component of strategic planning process. Most importantly, it requires knowledge about strategy, about different dimensions of performance, and how to establish performance targets, all of which will be described in this chapter.

PERFORMANCE IS MULTI-DIMENSIONAL

Hospitals and health systems exist for many obvious reasons, such as to heal the sick, improve the health of the community and research new treatments. Core services provided within healthcare organizations typically include observation, diagnosis, treatment and rehabilitation. Notice that these services revolve around patient and the public's health, which can be measured both clinically and medically. Quality measures and medical outcomes can be used to assess whether a health system did a reasonable job in these areas. Key questions to ascertain this assessment would include:

- Did the patient live?
- Did the patient make a full recovery?
- Did other complications arise during the patient's stay?

These types of questions have historically led the industry to measure outcomes in terms of two key metrics: mortality and morbidity. **Mortality** is a measure of the rate of incidence for deaths, whereas **morbidity** is a measure of the rate of illness. These are good macro-level indicators that reflect long-term efforts, but they are too broad to allow physicians and administrators to concentrate efforts on clinical improvements.

Consequently, many other more intermediate clinical outcomes and indicators that are linked to broad metrics are now being used to better measure performance. Metrics such as frequency of medical errors and incorrect filling of pharmaceutical prescriptions are two that are commonly used. We will discuss several others later in this chapter.

Yet healthcare involves more than medical outcomes. Healthcare organizations are expected to not only exist but to operate as a "going concern," and therefore, are expected to continue operations for the long term. This expectation suggests survival, and to survive long term, organizations must have controls over financial results—such as cash flows, margins, debt and working capital.

In the realm of financial results, outcome is dictated by how well operations and strategy perform. Operationally, factors such as the number of personnel, productivity, investment of information technology, space and facilities layout are all key to driving results. Strategically, organizations must focus on market share, growth rates, branding and other key outcomes. Quality metrics are just as important, such as clinical quality outcomes, as well as both service quality and patient satisfaction. Figure 2-1 shows how performance measures reflect long-term success in hospitals and health systems.

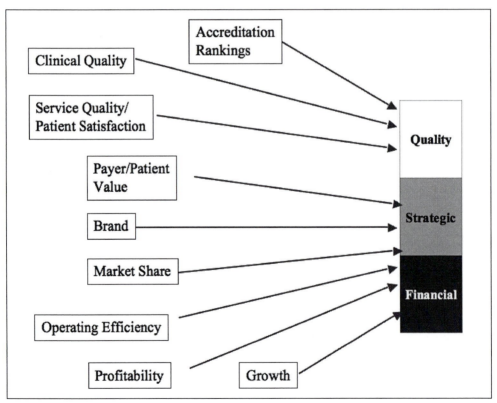

Figure 2-1: Health System Performance Is Multi-Dimensional

We have established that performance has multiple dimensions, all of which are important in different ways and times. As PI professionals typically focus on projects, the first task is to determine on which aspect of performance to focus our efforts. To determine this, we need a comprehensive framework for understanding the role of performance in healthcare.

HEALTHCARE STRATEGY AND PERFORMANCE FOR NON-PROFITS

The performance of a healthcare organization is typically measured by the extent to which it contributed toward the mission and vision of the organization. As most health systems and hospitals are not-for-profit, the mission is often stated in terms that are less about finances and more about serving the community, improving health outcomes and increasing service and clinical quality.

Many not-for-profit organizations base their purpose on a stated mission, which is typically defined in terms of meeting specific community needs. It is difficult, however, to hold them accountable for performance related to mission because specific metrics related to how well the mission is fulfilled are often neglected or difficult to measure. The performance measures that organizations are generally held to are often "means" objectives, as opposed to the mission "ends." For example, the mission often calls for an organization to provide health services that improve community health status and enhance quality of life; however, typical performance measures for which management is held accountable are generally such metrics as profitability, return on investment, market share and quality of care/service. Translating these to improvements in health status and quality of life might not be impossible but is certainly challenging. So the fundamental question to ask is how do society, boards and involved others hold organizations accountable for fulfilling their missions? How do we back into an assessment of how well management is doing with respect to mission and not just simply judge improvement according to the *means* measures of performance. To that end, we must move toward more direct measurement of "mission performance," so that we can evaluate an organization and its management in terms of how well they are doing with respect to their core purpose, i.e., the organization's mission. This will allow us to hold management and governance accountable for what they profess to be their purpose/mission. This is termed *mission accountability*.

With regard to mission accountability, there are three dimensions to measure:

1. How *much* an organization advances toward its stated mission (measures of quantity);
2. How *well* an organization does this (often termed *quality*); and
3. How efficiently the organization performs this aspect (cost-effectiveness).

If we integrate these three dimensions (quantity, quality and cost-effectiveness), we have a very good understanding of what healthcare organizations must do to thrive.

For most healthcare organizations, strategic performance can be seen as the sum of both mission performance and organizational performance, as shown in Figure 2-2.

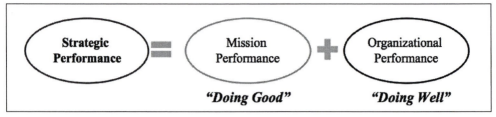

Figure 2-2: Strategic Performance

PERFORMANCE FRAMEWORK

In publicly traded industrial organizations, there is no dispute over goals and performance. Changes in market valuations and profitability (such as stock price, earnings per share and economic value added) are the dominant outcomes. All decisions are taken (at least theoretically under rational conditions) to maximize this key integrative performance metric. Because customer satisfaction, quality and operations need to be aligned to maximize even one of these metrics, and because these firms are attempting to maximize profits, these are very good for understanding the organization's overall health.

Hospitals and health systems, however, are different from other types of organizations in several respects, which make it difficult to apply one singular metric. Some of the differences are:

1. More than 85% of healthcare systems are not-for-profit in nature. Attempting to use financial performance as the outcome ignores the dominant mission.

2. Clinical and service quality often takes many years to become transparent to patients and payers. Although we are seeing many government agencies begin to push self-regulation and self-reporting of quality metrics, this trend is only in its infancy. Programs from both public and private organizations, such as the U.S. Department of Health and Human Services' Agency for Healthcare Research and Quality, The Joint Commission, the National Association for Healthcare Quality and the National Committee for Quality Assurance, are all making valuable strides toward quality reporting. Unfortunately, the transparency and visibility of these quality data, meanwhile have a lower impact on current performance than that of other industries.

3. Health systems are often required to take on charitable or indigent care, which obviously impacts financials significantly.

4. Healthcare organizations are aggressively investing in new medical technologies and research, which hopefully will pay off in terms of clinical outcomes in later years but which definitely has an impact on short-run performance.

Therefore, a useful performance framework for healthcare will not only integrate multiple aspects of financial performance, but will also outline a set of variables or indicators that will help to influence the other metrics. In Figure 2-3, a performance framework is presented.

Notice in this framework that each of the core dimensions of performance (i.e., quality, strategic/financial, operational and environmental) influence each other through bidirectional lines. That means all of these are related in one way or another. If you make changes in some, they impact others, either positively or negatively. Also,

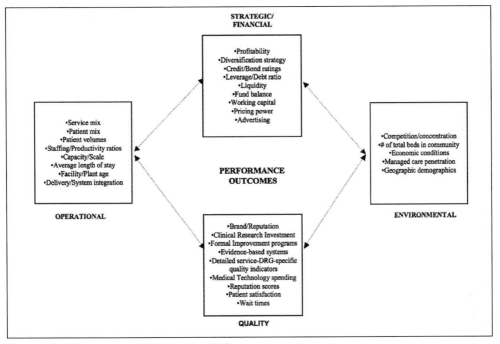

Figure 2-3: A Performance Model for Health Systems

the relative importance that each organization places on each dimension varies; some organizations focus most of their efforts on clinical quality, whereas others are focused on financials or operations. This choice of focus depends on a number of factors, such as their current state of affairs, the level of market turbulence or the phase of the organization's life cycle at which they are currently holding. Finally, notice the number of primary variables or indicators in each performance dimension, with many others that are not listed.

For every project that a management engineer or PI analyst undertakes, there *must* be a primary focus. Analysts should first ask themselves, and later ask the team this question: Which performance dimension is this project likely to positively impact? The first stage of process improvement or project management should start with either a prioritization or "business case," but in 9 of every 10 cases that we have reviewed, the measures of improvement are very qualitative, "soft" and intangible. Performance analysts must get to a deeper understanding of potential performance impacts prior to project kickoff, so the project can be mapped out with this in mind. Unfortunately, many healthcare organizations ignore this stage and later question why they did not realize any benefits.

Absent defined performance criterion, PI professionals should make their initial effort while focused on defining performance dimensions and specific key performance indicators and then ensuring that the project is managed to ultimately lead toward improvement in those areas. Figure 2-4 shows the link between upfront planning around performance impact and benefit realization.

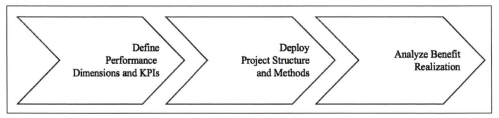

Figure 2-4: Benefit Realization Requires Performance Definition

CHANGE VERSUS IMPROVEMENT

All projects that a PI analyst or management engineer (ME) would undertake are in one of two forms: Either they are exploratory or they are change-oriented. In many cases however, even those descriptive or exploratory projects eventually become focused on change. In this context, descriptive or exploratory projects are those that simply seek to investigate current practices and describe existing processes. They are not focused on immediate change. **Change** is a transition from one state to another or a process of becoming different. Change is not always for the better, but it always results in things being different. Project professionals should *not* focus on achieving change for change sake but make improvement of indicators the focus of change. **Improvement** is positive change, or transition from something in a steady state to something better. Improvement adds value and delivers benefits in the expected performance dimension and specific key performance indicator (KPI).

As each project is undertaken, keeping the differences between change and improvement in mind is especially important. Projects, whether focused on process improvement or technology implementation, deliver change to people's work environments and processes. They may even impact their livelihood or that of their colleagues.

Improvement is relative. That is, improvement cannot become an absolute change across all projects for all measures. It must be defined in the initial project planning phase, with an understanding of the phase in which the existing performance currently exists, the level of resources and investment that will be made and the time frame provided. These three variables determine the relative improvements that can be made in any dimension.

STRATEGY AND PERFORMANCE

Performance improvement is tightly coupled with business strategy. Most healthcare organizations engage in a strategic planning process to develop a strategy or path to move from where they are today, to where they want to go. Both of these positions (current versus future) are measured in terms of performance, whether as market share, clinical quality, patient satisfaction or profitability. The mission of PI therefore is to enable strategy.

The process of achieving a strategy in healthcare is rarely as simple as one giant leap in a specific area; rather, it is a collection of small improvements in a number of domains. For example, if a hospital's primary strategy is to improve brand and competitive position, there may be a dozen or more initiatives that will have to be

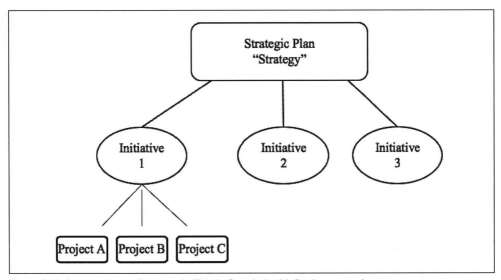

Figure 2-5: Organizational Strategy Is Tightly Coupled with Performance Improvement

developed to achieve the strategy. Figure 2-5 shows the relationship between strategy, initiatives and projects.

As this figure shows, improvements in a number of areas have to be made before strategic shifts can be seen in organizational performance. The process of setting performance objectives is typically one of the first processes in strategic planning. Many times, PI consultants working on a project might have their performance targets dictated to them as a result of the strategic plans. In other environments, the plans simply serve as the framework for setting priorities and target areas. Figure 2-6 shows a typical process of strategic planning and highlights the areas in which performance targets come into play.

PERFORMANCE-BASED PLANNING

Essentially, when improving an outcome is the desired impact, then all projects need to start with a performance-driven planning approach. This requires the management analyst or engineer to assemble the project team and clarify goals and objectives. Leading questions should be used, such as:

- Where are we trying to go? Where are we moving from?
- In which of the performance dimensions are we the weakest? The strongest?
- What are our competitors, or benchmark organizations doing in those areas? Are we falling behind them, or leading them?
- If we make a change in one performance area, will it affect other areas that we should be aware of now?
- How will these improvements affect patient satisfaction?
- Do we really know our current performance levels?
- Have we seen the measures graphically represented over time? Can we all agree on possible trends?

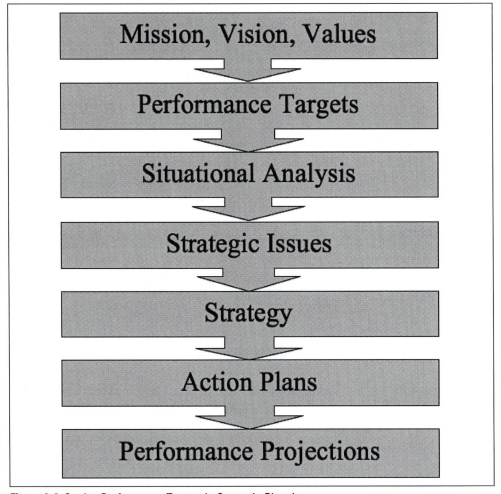

Figure 2-6: Setting Performance Targets in Strategic Planning

After these questions have been thoroughly explored, it becomes far easier to develop a common purpose for the project and to align the team around expectations and goals. This stage often takes considerable time, several hours per day for a week or longer—possibly more for really large projects, such as an enterprise resource planning (ERP) implementation.

Once these high-level plans are initiated, the management analyst needs to focus on performance specifics. These include asking questions, such as:

- What specific definition are we going to use for the metric? Although this may seem basic, it is necessary to apply a standardized and consistent definition to ensure comparability across other organizations and over time. The definition needs to be understood and embraced by all, so that it cannot be manipulated over the project to ensure project success.
- Where can we find existing data sources? What systems, either manual or electronic exist?
- If there are no existing sources of data, what investigational method will we use to measure current performance (e.g., pilot project to identify process costs, observe waiting times, collect quality indicators)?

- How long of a time period are we going to look backward and forward? A minimum of six months pre- and post- is normally of sufficient length, but many projects wish to look two or three years out.

Notice that all of this planning comes before a specific method or tool is even discussed. One of the common problems is that a PI analyst walks in the room with his Six Sigma toolkit or her "Plan-Do-Check-Act" (PDCA) methodology, but the first set of tasks is oriented toward discovery, not toward methods. **Discovery** is a thorough investigation of the present environment and collection of evidence. It requires that a thorough assessment be applied to understand performance relative to best practices. Once the discovery occurs, a method can be applied that is based on the unique goals and challenges brought forth in the discovery. Generally, one tool or method cannot be applied to all projects.

One of the most useful tools for discovery is the diagnostic assessment, which is custom created for each project. The assessment helps to quantitatively assess performance along a number of different process dimensions: personnel, technology, management systems, existing performance metrics and many others. It requires the ME to do some initial work to help research and catalog best practices for the specific process or department but is worth the trouble as it is invaluable to help prioritize work efforts and set the initial foundation. A sample diagnostic assessment for a generic process is seen in Figure 2-7.

Assessments such as these should be customized for each process and collectively evaluated by the group in order to provide project alignment and focus.

Best Practice/ Objective	Evaluation				
	1	2	3	4	5
1. Process has clear metrics and is routinely measured					
2. A technology plan exists for integrating the process					
3. Work is highly manual					
4. Participants understand the global (not just local) tasks					
5. Process trends are understood by administrators					
6. Productivity metrics are established and measurable					
7. Outsourcing is used as appropriate					
8. A contingency/backup system exists					
9. Staffing is aligned with demand					
10. Trends and metrics for accrued salaries are analyzed					
11. Employees are well trained in process					
12. There is a strong focus on customer service					
13. There is a strong focus on cycle time					
14. Errors and rework are measured and minimized					
15. Employees understand the direction and key goals					

Figure 2-7: Diagnostic Assessment Sample

SETTING PERFORMANCE TARGETS

Healthcare managers must find a way to define and align projects toward the performance dimensions, to enable the strategy. These dimensions could include automation and information systems, new building development, implementation of new service lines and many others. When the strategy has been established, the projects are defined, and the current performance levels are known, goals and objectives need to be established.

Although these two terms, goals and objectives are often used interchangeably, they are different. **Goals** are broad, long-term statements of an ideal future state. For instance, a very long-term goal would be "the elimination of diabetes." **Objectives,** on the other hand, are more specific, short-term, quantifiable statements that are readily measurable.

Goals and objectives help to transform the current performance level and path. With the introduction of a change (new project, system), the existing trend is shifted and results in new, hopefully more positive improvements in performance levels. Figure 2-8 shows this performance trajectory.

Whereas goals are typically broad and not easily measured on a periodic basis, objectives are more concrete and measurable on a periodic basis. Objectives represent specific targets for managers and PI analysts that should be tailored to individual projects. However, setting performance targets is often difficult. If the project manager sets goals that are too lofty, they become unachievable and may result in de-motivating staff and team members. If the goals are perceived as being too easy, they deliver only marginal value for the organization. Achieving the right balance is key, particularly where there are "stretch" goals that encourage positive change, deliver substantial value and motivate team members. Figure 2-9 shows the differences between goals and objectives and how levels impact the degree of difficulty involved.

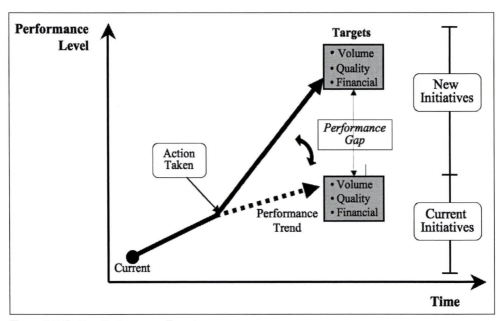

Figure 2-8: Setting Performance Targets

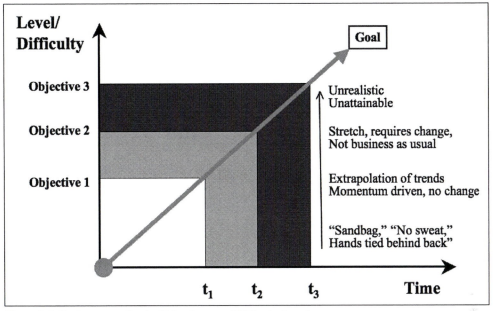

Figure 2-9: Performance Goals, Objectives, and Difficulty Levels

Also remember the guidelines for performance-based planning discussed earlier: performance targets must be measurable, quantifiable, consistent and reliable indicators over time for a particular performance dimension.

EXAMPLE: CASE STUDY

A project has been undertaken by the management of the operating room (OR) at Coles-Bart Regional Hospital, a mid-sized community hospital in urban Georgia, to improve their operations. The primary factors that initiated the project were patient complaints and a concern of OR management that the current capacity was insufficient to handle their daily demand of surgeries.

Lucy Bobs was assigned the role of project manager. Lucy, who is an industrial engineer by training, was assigned to the performance solutions department. Lucy's manager informed her that the OR was an especially "political" and influential realm of the hospital and that she needed to work very closely with them to ensure they remained satisfied.

Lucy assembled the team comprised of the OR administrator, a surgeon, a nurse manager and herself to assess the situation. She requested of the OR administrator access to the current performance metrics for the department and found there were no documented metrics in place. She was instructed to not let this "slow down progress" of the project. As a result. Lucy's first order was to have the team define an "ideal" environment, which would satisfy the participants. The team discussed and debated this question for some time and finally defined the ideal environment as one in which "patients move seamlessly through the perioperative period with no delays." This was promptly recorded as the core vision of the project.

The surgeon on the team, however, continued to offer his perspective that what the department needed was a new technology system called "OR Fantasy." This software would provide graphical reports that could be displayed in the hospital hallways and would therefore eliminate surgical rosters and manual schedules. He had seen the system in action at a recent conference. The system was discussed, competitive options were explored, and the vendor was called for pricing.

Soon thereafter, the purchasing department was contacted to put a request for a proposal (RFP) out, and after 60 more days, a license agreement was in place. Implementation began soon after, and "OR Fantasy" went live nearly 180 days later.

Following completion of the project, Lucy was asked to write a summary that explained and detailed the success of the project. She described the project as occurring over a duration of 250 days (well under the 365-day average project duration), having a rapid implementation of new technology and resulting in satisfied OR stakeholders. All in all, Lucy considered this a highly successful project!

In this case study, the industrial engineer did a good job helping to keep momentum strong among team members, achieving some level of perceived success (the decided ideal environment), and keeping the team intact, which is sometimes quite a feat. However, many lessons can be learned about what Lucy failed to do properly. She failed to perform benchmarking functions, she allowed the primary sponsor (surgeon) to direct the efforts solely toward a technology solution and she allowed the project to be defined too narrowly in terms of expectations. All of these can be overcome by following the guidelines and suggestions offered next.

BENCHMARKING

One way to establish benefit or performance targets is to *benchmark* the same targets against other comparable hospitals or health systems. **Benchmarking** is the comparison of a key performance measurement relative to that of the competition or other leading organizations.[1] It can also be defined as the process of seeking best practices among better performing organizations, with intentions of applying those practices internally.

There are a number of types of benchmarking—those that focus on process, services, best practices or competition. Although their specific focus or unit of analysis is different, in most respects, the purpose of each type is the same (to compare and assess), For example, suppose there are five hospitals in the same large, urban city. A performance engineer has been hired by the chief nursing officer to help analyze how overall nursing productivity (measured as the number of total procedures performed divided by the nursing labor time) compares with the other four organizations. At a high level, the engineer could simply look up the labor and volume data historically, using secondary published data available from the American Hospital Directory or the American Hospital Association. Doing this provides a baseline comparison that can be analyzed over time to enable an observation of trends. This example of *competitive benchmarking* is one in which the best practice organizations can be identified and further reviewed. If the engineer were to phone the other sites, ask for a walk-through of the floors or units and observe the functions in detail, this would be a good example of *process benchmarking*.

There are limitations and advantages to using either primary or secondary data in benchmarking. Obviously, the use of direct interviews and observation is typically better than using secondary data, as the data are more real-time and allow for feedback and communication about definitions and metrics. However, primary data also have their own limitations, such as when the interviewee provides biased or skewed responses based on his or her interpretation of questions or when attempting to make his or her process appear superior to others.

The best way we have found to collect performance benchmarking data is to use best-practice organizations in other locales to avoid competitive concerns about sharing data. The process is fairly straightforward, having only five steps: (1) identify problems and gaps; (2) identify best practice organizations; (3) prepare for site visit; (4) conduct site visit; and (5) adopt practices into your organization.

Identify Problems and Gaps

Identify your organization or department's specific problem area, whether it is a process concern or a performance gap. Clearly document the problem, and define current process capabilities. These include analysis of the historical data and trends and the use of a capability index (such as C_{pk}, described in the next chapter), using statistical analyses of the transactional or performance data when possible.

Research and Identify Best Practice Organizations

Using newsletters, journals, magazines or case studies and library searches, conduct a search of those organizations that appear to have best practice, organizations that have established themselves as leaders in the specific area on which you are focusing. Once identified, the organizations are contacted and site visits requested. Other potential resources for data include the following associations, organizations and agencies:
- Healthcare Information and Management Systems Society (www.himss.org)
- American College of Healthcare Executives (www.ache.org)
- Healthcare Financial Management Association (www.hfma.org)
- American Medical Informatics Association (www.amia.org)
- National Association for Healthcare Quality (www.nahq.org)
- Centers for Medicare & Medicaid Services (www.cms.hhs.gov)
- The Joint Commission (www.jointcommission.org)
- U.S. News and World Report (http://health.usnews.com)
- American Hospital Directory (www.ahd.com)
- American Hospital Association (www.aha.org)
- ProQuest ABI/Inform (www.proquest.com)
- National Institute for Health and Clinical Excellence, UK (www.nice.org.uk)

Prepare for Benchmarking Visit

Prepare detailed plans for what you hope to gain from these visits. Preparation is key and is often minimized. Adequate preparation ensures that a full set of questions is developed, a plan for the time spent with the host is constructed and shared and both parties understand the goals and objectives for the visit. Showing up at a benchmarking site without a plan is a waste of resources. Questions will obviously vary by site and by process. For an evaluation of a new information system, for which best practices of the implementation are to be analyzed, some generic questions could include the following:

- What was the projected benefit versus the amount realized? What was the primary reason for the variance?
- Which one system drives most of the business value?
- What is an estimate of the total cost of the implementation? What portion of this cost was planned versus unexpected?
- What are some of the biggest lessons learned?
- If you could do the implementation over again, what would you do differently?
- What are you least proud about the implementation?
- Which task on the project timeline took significantly more time or resources than you estimated? How many people were involved in the overall project? How many were 100% dedicated?
- Which vendors did you select? Why were they chosen?
- What was the total project timeline? Was it far off from the original projection?
- What was the overall reaction by your staff in the beginning (e.g., positive, negative, indifferent)? What explains these views?
- What were the three greatest improvements in actual performance indicators or process capabilities?
- Were there any technical or system glitches of which we should be aware?
- What surprises were encountered?
- What role did consultants play in this process?
- Can we see an example of the system?
- Do you have any performance scorecards we can examine?

Conduct Site Visit

The next step is to conduct the actual site visit, executing the materials prepared from the previous step, specifically being sure to have all the questions addressed so that you understand the best practice and are able to adopt it post-benchmarking. It is important to bring the right people to the visit and assign one in the group to take detailed notes and collect any documentation necessary for follow-up. During the visit, it is critical to observe first-hand the participants, events, activities and systems in the process being reviewed.

Adopt and Integrate Best Practices

Post-visit, it is important to gather the benchmarking team to discuss findings, document the best practices observed and, most importantly, immediately incorporate these into plans and process changes to be implemented. Adapting the best practices and adopting them into your own plan is the only way that benchmarking proves to be a valuable exercise.

GUIDELINES FOR PERFORMANCE MANAGEMENT

Following are five guidelines for PI consultants to use to deliver value to the organization.

Define Success More Carefully

One of the most common problems in process improvement work is that the initial task of defining desired performance is often cut short. Healthcare administrators tend to believe they already know the problems that exist and how they plan to proceed, without careful analysis or discovery of facts. More than any other industry, healthcare tends to define performance very abstractly and broadly, which makes it easy to claim success in post-project evaluations but very difficult to prove.

In this case study, the initial effort that was needed should have been to select a performance dimension and associated set of KPIs from the beginning. Collaboratively, the group needed to spend an appropriate amount of time brainstorming and planning desired performance impacts: Would a project impact quality, financials, operations or a combination? Using which specific metric? In many cases, there has been virtually no planning around performance indicators; therefore, when a project for technology or process is initiated, the first step is always to carefully plan! It is easy to skip this step, but then all that a project can claim is that it has delivered change, not improvement.

Measure Historical Performance

In general, once a team identifies the ideal performance criteria, development of a methodology for collecting and analyzing the data behind that indicator is needed. In our earlier project description, assume one criterion, waiting times for patients, for example, was improved. Without an understanding of current levels of wait periods, how can an organization suggest that any improvements were made post-project? Unfortunately, that is what happens in many cases: Organizations claim they do not have the right system or process in place to measure current results; therefore, only after the project is successful can they begin to measure. This is flawed thinking.

In industrial organizations, only those projects that have the potential to deliver results are undertaken. To prove results, a measure of the delta, or change, between pre- and post-project metrics must be taken. This discipline must become more customary in healthcare if real improvements are to be made. Industrial engineers, project managers and PI professionals all play a pivotal role in helping make this measurement a reality.

Forecast Desired Improvement Target

Once the performance indicator is established and historic data are collected, the team must create a target to establish direction and level for that criterion. If the target is improved waiting times, and historically the OR includes 1.6 hours of wait pre-surgery, the project needs a reasonable target for future performance. Ideally, the new target should be staged, based on timing. An example is, "in the first six months post-project, wait times will decrease 30% to 67 minutes." The desired performance target now becomes:

- *Measurable*, in both absolute and relative terms;
- *Quantitative*, using precise percentage changes numerically;
- *Consistent*, with existing definition and data over multiple periods; and
- *Relevant*, by using the right performance dimension.

More about setting performance targets will be described in Chapter 3.

Remember, the PI Analyst Is the Expert!

As the project professional, it is up to you to ensure that the project achieves the right result—that is, the group follows a methodology, consistently applies rigor and ensures that projects focus on results, outcomes and positive change. As the expert, the PI analyst must use his or her authority to guide the project in the right direction over the long run.

In larger organizations, politics or bureaucracy will always impede progress. However, if the PI analyst does the right thing, is trained in the right methodology, is diligent about results and facilitates effectively, "impeding" will not lead to "preventing" project success.

Don't Let Benefits Leak Out

Performance gains do accrue, but even those projects that are meticulously planned and executed have some benefit leakage. According to Mankins and Steele,[2] only 63% of the total potential performance gains are realized by most organizations. Performance losses occur because of inadequate resources, poor strategy, lack of accountability, lack of monitoring and for many other reasons. Using the right methods for the right project and maintaining a perspective focused on pre- and post-performance is key to maintaining performance gains over the long term.

SUMMARY

Performance is multi-dimensional. Health systems are here to survive, provide valuable services to the community and improve patient outcomes, among other reasons. Performance improvement engineers are often tasked with leading projects. A critical (but often overlooked) step in leading such a charge is to carefully define performance criteria before undertaking the project. Benefits can never be realized from a project or process change if initial performance planning does not occur and if precise performance measures are not collected for the past and projected into the future.

References

1. Langabeer JR. *Healthcare Operations Management: A Quantitative Approach to Business and Logistics.* Boston: Jones and Bartlett Publishers; 2007.
2. Mankins MC, Steele R. Turning great strategy into great performance. *Harvard Business Review.* 2005; 83:64-72.

CHAPTER 3

Metric Identification and Benefit Realization

Cynthia McKinney

> *"Always produce more than you promise."*
> — Richard Nixon, former U.S. President

INTRODUCTION

In healthcare today, a benefit is always anticipated when an organization engages in a new service or technology. The benefit may be a gain in market share, improved patient safety, reduced costs or improved productivity. However, many organizations do not implement a process for identifying metrics and measuring the benefit because either it is not seen as a priority or it lacks executive support or buy-in. As a result, many organizations are often unable to fully understand or quantify the benefit of their efforts.

This chapter provides an introduction to metrics and benefits. Topics include: the strategy and approach organizations should consider; steps for identifying metrics and gathering baseline data; activities for establishing targets; an overview for developing a monthly process; and discussion of the key components for ongoing measurement and monitoring of the results.

METRICS AND BENEFITS

The terms *metrics* and *benefits* imply different things to different organizations. Metrics are common in healthcare—for example, average length of stay, days in accounts receivable or nursing hours per patient day. Metrics are used to track both financial and operational performance, as well as in regulatory reporting, such as that performed by the Centers for Medicare & Medicaid Services (CMS) or The Joint Commission. Benefits, on the other hand, may be only an afterthought of a process. Although organizations are interested and have a stake in knowing the value they will receive for large investments, they do not consistently identify the appropriate metrics or implement the process to track the benefit.

Metrics can be identified and used to measure benefits within all levels of an organization (e.g., service line executives, vice presidents and department managers). The audience for each set of metrics and benefits will vary based on the specific metrics and purpose for each.

Although metrics and benefits are quite different terms, they are frequently confused. A contrast of the definitions follows in Table 3-1.

Table 3-1: Metrics and Benefits

Term	Wikipedia	Commonly Used Definition
Metric	A **metric** is a standard unit of measure, such as mile or second, or more generally, part of a system of parameters, or systems of measurement, or a set of ways of quantitatively and periodically measuring, assessing, controlling or selecting a person, process, event, or institution, along with the procedures to carry out measurements and the procedures for the interpretation of the assessment in the light of previous or comparable assessments. Metrics are usually specialized by the subject area, in which case they are valid only within a certain domain and cannot be directly benchmarked or interpreted outside it.	A metric is a measurement that includes a distinct numerator and denominator developed specifically to measure the established goal or objective.
Benefit	**Benefit** may refer to: Something that a party was not previously entitled to receive. Economic benefit, the positive contribution to gross national product (or other measure of value) from an economic activity or project.	The benefit is the perceived value that will be achieved with the new service or technology. The benefit will be measured by the identified metrics.

Source: Wikipedia, 2008.

Useful to this discussion are clear breakouts of key terms. Benefit realization, for example, is the process and guideline for measuring and ensuring that a project or program delivers expected performance benefits (e.g., stated goals). The key steps for benefit realization—developing and implementing successful metrics—are presented in Figure 3-1. Each step is further defined in the sections that follow.

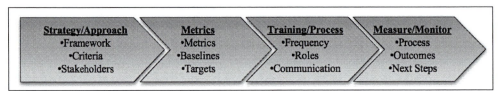

Figure 3-1: Metric Implementation Process

STRATEGY AND APPROACH

Prior to identifying the actual metrics that will be used, several strategic questions must be answered. These questions will aid in framing the process.

How Will the Metrics Be Used?

An organization must decide how the metric will be used, for instance, whether it will be part of routine operations or only used for executive dashboard reporting. This decision will help drive the type of metrics to develop.

Consideration must be given to the duration of the metrics, specifically, if it is to be short or long term or if it will become an ongoing measure within the organization.

Who Is Driving the Metrics Process?

An organization must think through how it will gain organization buy-in to the identified metrics and process. Making it CXO or board-driven alone does not guarantee that the user community will embrace the process. The process must include all key stakeholders from day one through the end of the project. In addition, all aspects of a project must be communicated to steering committees on an on-going basis.

Who Are the Users/Stakeholders?

Unfortunately, this key question is often overlooked. It is critical to identify the stakeholders and involve them early in the process. Whereas the executive staff of an organization must develop the strategic framework, the operational stakeholders must be a part of the process from day one to gain buy in. The stakeholders will be defined differently based on the type of organization; for example, if the organization is a multi-hospital organization, consideration should be given to whether the metrics will be consistently applied to all stakeholders.

In addition to these three questions, the following four questions should also be addressed to provide a detailed framework for accurately identifying the metrics. To maximize the process, these questions should be answered *before* beginning the metrics identification phase.

What Are the Data Requirements for the Metrics?

Each organization must identify its unique guidelines for metrics, using questions such as: Will baseline data be required? How much historical data will be required? If the data collection process is complex, will we continue?

Do the Metrics Need to Be Financially Quantifiable?

The decision whether financially quantifiable metrics are required must be identified at the beginning of the project, as it will impact the metrics identification process.

How Many Metrics Should Be Selected?

The number of metrics chosen should be manageable and worth the time spent during the development process and on-going measurement. Suggested guidelines for small projects recommend between 3 and 5 metrics; larger implementations might have between 10 and 12 metrics and systemwide initiatives should have no more than 20 metrics.

What Is the Desired Reporting Frequency?

Reporting should occur as frequently as possible, given the availability and accessibility of the data. This should be based on the defined need around frequency of reporting (e.g., daily real time, monthly, quarterly).

METRICS—IDENTIFICATION, VALIDATION, BASELINES AND TARGETS

The most important step in the process is to identify the appropriate metrics. Although there are many considerations, the most critical component is to *develop the metrics that support the goals and initiatives of the project*. This seemingly easy statement is the most difficult part of the project. The following sections outline key considerations of the metrics identification process.

Metrics Identification

In applying the framework developed from the strategy and approach section previously discussed, an organization should have adequate guidelines with which to develop metrics. One of the first questions addresses how to define metrics to support the project.

Key to developing correct metrics is linking the metrics to the project goals and objectives. For each project goal, there may be more than one objective, and for each objective there may be several metrics. Therefore, it is critical that the goals and objectives are fully understood before beginning this process.

An example of this process is shown in Table 3-2. (Note that many metrics may be applied and the following is an example for illustrative purposes only.)

Table 3-2: Sample Project Metrics

Project Goals	Project Objectives	Example Metrics
Patient safety	Reduce medication errors through electronic medication administration record (eMAR)	• Transcription errors rate
Clinical quality and patient safety	Improve efficient outcomes	• Care guideline rate of use by care plan • Clinical practitioner order entry (CPOE) utilization rate
Patient safety	Reduce turnaround times	• Turnaround time for lab results • Turnaround time for results reporting
Cost containment	Reduce labor costs	• Surgery labor cost per case • Labor cost per FTE

Metric Development Process

Based on the purpose of the metrics, an organization may need to develop metrics for different audiences. A common separation of metrics includes:

- Multi-facility corporate executives—metrics that enable a cross-entity comparison;
- Hospital-based executives—metrics that enable a single facility to understand their financial and operational change; and
- Department managers—metrics that enable department managers to better understand the impact on their departments.

An organization may develop metrics for any or all of the audiences. An example of the types of metrics is shown in Table 3-3.

Securing Organizational Buy-In

Gaining organization buy-in has proven to be highly challenging for many organizations. The following approaches should be considered:

- Ensure that stakeholders are involved from the beginning, as well as in all other phases of the process—not just during the metric identification phase.
- Draft a lengthy list of potential metrics, and have the stakeholders identify the final metrics to be used.
- Assign the metrics to the individual stakeholders accountable for tracking progress.

Metric Definition Process

Often seen as a simple task, preparing the definition for the metrics can present quite a challenge. The following guidelines should be considered during this process:

1. Clearly document the definition. For example:
   - Appointment or case cancellation/changes rate – patient request: the number of times appointments or cases are rescheduled or cancelled at the request of the patient.
2. Clearly document the calculation. For example:
   - (Number of appointments or cases changed or cancelled at the request of the patient / number of appointments) × 100.
3. Document both what is included, as well as what is excluded from the definition:
   - The proposed metric appointment or case cancellations/change rate – patient request excludes appointments cancelled by the physician or department.
4. Document the source of the metric:
   - The source of the metric must be identified for both baseline (existing) data, as well as for the future source of the metric. Clear documentation will identify potential discrepancies in the calculations and will assist during the audit process.
5. Consider how this definition may vary from other existing calculations of the same metric. For example, the finance department may measure the same metric but in a slightly different way. Close consideration and synchronization of the metrics must occur.
6. Do not expend effort on developing a variation of current metrics if not necessary.

7. Consider all metrics of an organization. Healthcare organizations are required to track many items, and the last thing you want to do is to add nonmeaningful metrics.

Table 3-3: Metrics by Audience Type

Type of Metric/ Metric Name	Multi-Facility Corporate Executives	Hospital Executives	Department Managers
Financial			
Inpatient cost per discharge	•	•	
Financial summary to budget	•	•	•
Labor or supply cost per visit	•	•	•
Medication cost per case		•	•
Net income	•	•	
Operational			
Average length-of-stay days	•		
Number of patient days or discharges	•	•	
Patient wait times (e.g., scheduling / ED)		•	•
Employee turnover rate	•	•	•
Lost film rate			•
Nursing hours per patient day		•	•
Clinical Quality			
Adverse drug event rate	•	•	•
Mortality rate	•	•	
Nursing medication administration time			•
Order change rate		•	•
Regulatory measures (e.g., CMS, The Joint Commission)	•	•	•
Marketing (Front-End Required Data)			
Number of referrals—by site/facility, payer	•	•	
Disease specific outcomes compliance rate			•
Percent referrals by provider/physician	•	•	
Service/Performance			
Physician order entry rate	•	•	
Pre-registration rate			•
Patient, physician, staff satisfaction rate	•	•	•
Discharge processing time			•
Process efficiency rate (specific productivity reporting)		•	•

Metrics Validation

The validation of the proposed metrics is a two-step process. You must validate not only acceptance of the metrics with the stakeholders but also that the definition and calculation are accurate:

1. Stakeholder validation. All key stakeholders should review the metrics to ensure they understand and support how the metric will support their initiative. Key to this process is stakeholders' understanding of why this metric was selected and how this metric will support the benefit of measuring the new service or technology.

2. Definition and calculation validation. Validate the calculations and definitions with the stakeholders. Ensure that the results of the proposed metrics provide the expected results.

METRICS BASELINE MEASUREMENT

Although recommended, baseline measures are not required. However, they *are* required to validate the metrics, as well as to establish target improvement ranges and show improvement and progress. The key components of baseline measurements include addressing the following issues:

1. What is the amount of data required for baseline measures?
   - The recommended amount of data to calculate the baseline is between 3 and 6 months of data. It is important that you select a period of time that will provide an accurate reflection of the change. The timeframe for the baseline data should be consistent for all metrics.

2. Who collects the baseline data?
   - The baseline collection process can be quite labor intensive. It should be collected and validated by those who are familiar with data and data calculations.
   - Many organizations bypass this step due to the intense labor of the effort.

3. What are the data sources for the baseline data?
   - The data sources must be explicitly defined. This includes where the data are being pulled from (which system), the criteria and detailed definitions of the calculations and the definitions of the data.
   - If the data are not available, an organization must decide if it will forego baseline measures or if it should collect data immediately and use a shorter time period.

4. What is done once the baseline data are collected?
   - The baseline data must be collected and compiled into a format that reflects the proposed metric calculations. This will allow the required comparison with the post-implementation results in order to determine the amount of change.
   - The baseline data will also provide the basis for establishing targets (see the next section).

METRICS TARGETS AND GOALS

As described in Chapter 2, establishing targets and goals is highly recommended but not always completed. The creation of targets will allow an organization to calculate the benefits it expects to receive. To calculate the benefits, both the baselines and targets (or goals) must be collected.

Difference between Targets and Goals

Although the terms targets and goals are often used interchangeably, there is a slight difference in meaning. A goal is the improvement amount the organization is trying to achieve (e.g., reduce costs by 5%). A target reflects the actual value the organization is trying to achieve (e.g., reduce costs by a goal of 5%, resulting in a target value of $35.50).

Target/Goal Setting

The most objective way to set a target or goal is to conduct industry research to identify the best practice or optimum operating levels. The research will provide a combination of both goals and targets, which will then need to be interpreted to the data set being used. When using industry data, it is recommended that a minimum of five articles be reviewed to support the recommendation.

How Are Targets Used to Quantify the Benefit?

The targets (or goals) are used to calculate the percent savings. The benefit amount can be calculated by applying the target value to projected volume to estimate the projected benefit. It requires the following:

- Identified metric (with clear calculation);
- Baseline data—quantified in terms of dollars;
- Targets or goals;
- Projected volume (as related to the metric); and
- Applying the target or goals to the baseline data, so the benefit amount can be estimated.

PROCESS AND TRAINING

Although much time is spent on defining metrics and calculating benefits, just as important is the need to define the process for how the metrics will be reported and validated. Once defined, an organization is ready to complete the training and initiate the process.

1. What should be defined in the process?
   - The process should cover *who*, *when*, and *how* metrics are reported.
     Who—Define *who* will report the results (if manual), *who* will validate the results for reasonableness, and *who* will compile the results.
       If the process is fully automated, the information still requires validation, which needs to be defined.
       If the metric reporting is for a healthcare system, the process for all facilities must be defined (e.g., centralized reporting and validation).
     When—Define *when* the results will be reported. For example, will all data be required to be submitted the last day of the month? Or, the tenth day of

the month? Bear in mind that the reporting timeframe must be the same for all metrics to ensure consistency.

How—Define *how* the results will be compiled, reported and acted on. It is recommended that a dashboard report be created. If an organization currently maintains a dashboard, the metrics may be appropriate to roll into the same reporting structure and format.

2. Who is responsible for what?
   - Responsibilities must be clearly defined to ensure accountability and follow-through for the following roles: accountable individual/stakeholder, manual reporting, compilation/reporting, results review and action plan.
3. Who needs to be trained?
   - Following the process and roles definition, all affected individuals should be trained, preferably through both written and presentation material.

MEASURING AND MONITORING

When the reporting process actually begins, there are additional steps that must be taken to validate the results, as well as actionable steps needed to respond to the results.

1. How often should the results be verified?
   - The reporting and results should be verified monthly for the first six months and then quarterly thereafter.
2. How often should the results be reviewed by management?
   - All managers—specifically the stakeholders—should review the results on a monthly basis. They need to be prepared to complete the executive reporting, which should occur at least quarterly.
3. What executive reporting should be completed?
   - To ensure that monitoring is performed, executive reporting should occur at least quarterly and should include a project status update, summary of savings, status on achieving targets, critical issues preventing benefits realization and additional opportunities.

SUMMARY

When an organization wants to ensure it achieves benefits from its investment, there must be upfront planning, thought and effort to develop all aspects of the program. Thinking through the details—such as the type of metric, definitions, development processes, buy-in, change management and other details—will help to ensure benefit realization. Although the process itself is not difficult, it is time-consuming, involves substantial analytical and communication skills and requires buy-in at all levels of the organization.

SECTION II

GOVERNING PERFORMANCE IMPROVEMENT PROGRAMS

It is nearly impossible for management engineers to improve performance without the use of structure and methods—governance, to be precise. The way in which PI is organized, managed and evaluated establishes the degree of success the group is going to achieve. In Section II we discuss the steps necessary to create a new organization that is focused on PI, how best to manage the organization (including the selection of projects and monitoring of results), the basics of process redesign and project management and how to continuously improve the visibility and significance of the PI department.

In Chapter 4, Rigoberto Delgado (a senior management engineer at a leading medical center) and I discuss how to best establish and lead a PI department, a pertinent topic as there recently has been a resurgence of energy around PI, and many new teams are being developed. We discuss project intake and evaluation methods with a focus on maximizing outcomes for your project portfolio, and aligning the right methods to these projects. We then focus on unique ways to show the value and concepts that act as foundations for management engineering groups.

In Chapter 5, Rigoberto Delgado and I discuss the basics of both change and project management. Project success is often only achieved when the engineer develops "softer" skills—such as communication and facilitation; and understanding these qualitative aspects of a project is usually as important as having an understanding of the technical components. We also provide some insight into how to avoid common pitfalls in dealing with organizational change.

In Chapter 6, Kim Brant-Lucich, a former management consultant and now a leading authority on process redesign at a large California health system, describes the framework for process redesign. She discusses how to incorporate process improvement techniques into system implementations and the basics of assessing problems, identifying solutions and engaging stakeholders in the solutions.

CHAPTER 4

Managing Process Improvement

James Langabeer II and Rigoberto Delgado

> *"Quality is everyone's responsibility."*
>
> — W. Edwards Deming

INTRODUCTION

Formally organizing a department that focuses on improving processes is very difficult for many reasons. First, few completely new departments or units are created each year. While most hospitals and systems have some form of a decision support or PI department in place, most of these departments are small and are focused on specific areas of the organization. Second, gaining the approval and support of executives, as well as the resource commitment for staff and other expenses, is typically a lengthy and time-consuming process in itself. Finally, new departments challenge the status quo and, without strong leadership from a sponsor or champion, tend to fall by the wayside. Even when you have gained ME or PI team approval, the challenges do not stop there. This chapter outlines guidelines for establishing and leading such an effort.

STEPS TOWARD BUILDING A PERFORMANCE IMPROVEMENT DEPARTMENT

In a large teaching hospital at which one of us had served in senior leadership, the need arose for the development of a team that could apply analytical methods to improve decisions, plans and processes. For many years, the hospital had operated a department that focused on clinical quality and PI initiatives. But for such a large and complex organization—with approximately 16,000 employees and nearly 600 beds—there was a growing need to evaluate operational effectiveness in other areas, namely the business and support service areas. Despite the large amount of resources available, this large hospital suffered from what can be referred to as "silo" structures, and, consequently, each division primarily relied on its own staff for improvements.

In November 2005, under the direction of the chief financial officer, a management engineering and analysis department was created. The initial scope of the department was a focus on the areas of finance and supply chain but was later expanded to include significant efforts around information systems, business planning, project management and facilities development. Following are the steps we followed to develop the initial concept that would serve as the basis for a new department of ME.

Develop Concept/Position

The first step in the process of creating a new department must be to develop a thorough concept or position to be used as a model. This concept details potential benefits, risks, costs and a vision for the functions of the department. Identifying how the mission or purpose is different from any other department in the current organization structure is key to differentiating it from other functions. Typically, most PI departments focus on the following areas:

- Project management, such as that found in large systems, facility development or others
- Process improvement, of clinical and support processes
- Decision support, analytics and modeling for decision making and planning
- Performance management, including benchmarking and scorecard development
- Information technology assessment, implementation and evaluation
- Operational and business planning

Create Business Case/Proposal

The next step is to convert the concept into a proposal that can be exchanged and discussed at multiple levels of the organization. This proposal should contain traditional aspects of all proposals, such as discussion of benefits, business drivers, benchmarks and resource requirements. Figure 4-1 suggests a format for the business case.

Sponsorship/Champion	•Identify the project sponsor and champion
Business Drivers/Vision	•Describe the challenges on which the department should focus •Identify benefit areas •Describe how these opportunities impact performance and contribute to the organization's vision •Describe the division to which the department will report
Benefits/Outcomes	•Describe the key performance indicators (KPI) and how the department could impact specific indicators •Document outcomes expectations and improvement areas •Monetarize the "value" of these outcomes over time
Benchmarks	•If possible, outline competitive organizations and their use of similar PI units •Describe implications on organization, policy and processes
Investment/Resource Requirements	•Define the proposed investment in terms of staffing, space, technology •Define recommendations for moving forward •List all key assumptions •Document the risks and how they can be mitigated •Define timelines and key milestones

Figure 4-1: Proposing a New PI Department

In order to correctly prepare this proposal, the human resource (HR) components will need to be defined early on, as HR costs will likely consume 75% or more of the operating budget. Meetings with HR should outline organizational development, skill profiles of talent (PI professionals), compensation requirements and a general recruiting strategy. Key skills for PI professionals will need to incorporate strong internal consulting background, project management, facilitation, change management and knowledge of information systems, a combination of skills that is often difficult to find in a single person.

The intricacies of structure in relation to reporting relationships can represent a tricky situation. Typically, in larger organizations, there are multiple departments in large divisions focused on project management, process improvement and decision support. These groups can represent barriers and competition, or they can serve as sources of partnership and collaboration. Deciding how to incorporate them into the vision and concept is critical from the beginning.

Another challenge for many organizations is deciding where to locate the PI department. Of course, most PI managers would prefer reporting to the CEO, but research shows this is very rare.[1] In many cases, the new department resides within the Information Systems department. In other organizations, it is embedded in Clinical Operations, Finance or Nursing departments. These are not standard models for success and ways of structuring reporting relationships; however, PI departments can thrive under any of these, as long as they follow the other recommendations that follow.

Gain Executive Consensus and Support

Unless you are the CEO or chairman of the board of trustees, the necessary next step, once the proposal has been developed, will be to build support. In some organizations, this step involves simply going up one level in the organization and asking for approval. But in most organizations today, this step requires garnering support from a variety of executives throughout the organization. In our case, all of the key executives were given an opportunity to hear the business proposal and offer suggestions. This process of *pre-wiring,* as it is called, allows stakeholders to provide input, which can be incorporated into subsequent revisions. When these sessions are conducted offline and not in groups, everybody benefits, and it does not jeopardize the approval process.

In striving to build support by describing need, one of the more difficult executives to convince is typically the chief financial officer (CFO), a fact that makes evident the importance of clearly outlined investment (costs, resources) stated in "value" terms, so that costs can be compared with gains. Most CFOs prefer to use net present value (NPV) or other similar time value of money concepts to ensure that total benefits exceed total costs. Doing this in advance of their review and being certain to outline all assumptions are very important.

In total, the idea of *selling* the concept often takes several months and requires continuous motivation and discipline to move to the next step.

Rollout Phases

Once approval and support have been gained, the rollout or initiation can begin. As no organization can jump from non-existence to full operation, it is important to use

Phase 1	Phase 2	Phase 3
•Recruit management •Develop vision •Begin identifying initial project(s)	•Define/Adopt methodology •Form toolkit of methods •Recruit staff •Educate team •Begin communication and marketing efforts •Share initial results/gains	•Develop project assessment/intake criteria •Develop project scorecard •Further integrate department into institutional processes

Figure 4-2: Phased-in Approach to PI Development

a phased-in approach, which typically refers to an incremental strategy, gradually showing value over time.

In the first phase, the vision and mission of the department are developed, as well as recruitment of the key manager for the group. Since recruiting can take between three and twelve months, depending on location and other factors, this first phase can often take as long as a year or even longer. In creating the ME department as our case study, we chose an initial vision as helping the institution "...discover value opportunities" and using "advanced methods to transform processes and performance throughout the organization."

In the second phase, additional staff must be recruited and educated, methodologies developed or adopted and toolkits of methods collected. In large institutions, communication efforts, or marketing, also will need to occur to offset the possibility of lack of visibility. E-mail distributions, announcements and/or brown-bag seminars to share results of the department's initial projects are necessary for achieving wider integration into the organization. In the final stage, as more projects are requested by departments and other user groups, a process for project intake will have to be developed. Another chapter will more fully discuss this topic. Figure 4-2 shows the phases of development for a new ME or PI department.

MANAGING PERFORMANCE IMPROVEMENT

Managing PI or ME teams is a process of managing groups of internal consultants with a portfolio of projects in various stages. In the early phase of developing a new department, the focus of management should be on selecting and educating the right individuals and then selecting the initial set of methodologies to be used. It is important that PI managers align their organizational context with the project management framework. Careful understanding of the organization's strategies, players and current performance drivers will dictate specific methods, intake or evaluation processes and other aspects of projects. Figure 4-3 presents the suggested alignment between organizational and project environments.

What to Look for in a PI Professional

Recruiting and hiring MEs are often difficult. The quality of the mix of skills, education and previous experience is vital. During the formative years, it is important to recruit individuals eager to build and adapt, because structure and methods will not exist from day one. Flexibility is a key skill, although it is difficult to measure.

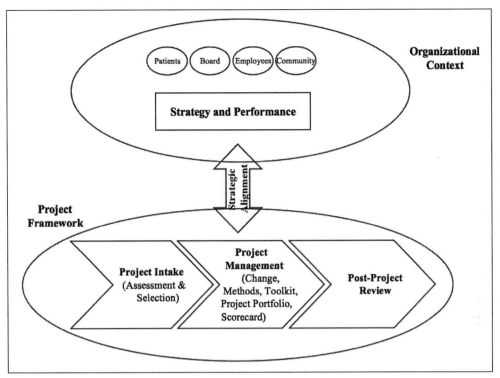

Figure 4-3: Performance Improvement Framework

No two PI consultants have the same educational background. In earlier years a candidate with an industrial engineering degree would have been optimal, given that course of study's focus on understanding systems concepts and processes; now, however, most analysts will have business, nursing, information technology, allied health or numerous other degrees. An undergraduate degree requirement is common for this position in most organizations.

A candidate with a background in internal or external consulting is also ideal. The ability to understand internal customers (often called *user groups*), facilitate project meetings and creative sessions and listen to clients to understand the symptoms of larger problems is required. In short, the following skills are necessary:

- Diagnostic capabilities
- Combination of engineering (technical) and organizational development (soft) skills
- Project management
- Customer service
- Communication
- Knowledge of enterprise information systems, databases and applications
- Systems modeling
- Use of analytical tools

Methodology

One of the critical tasks for an emerging department is to choose the right methodology. Among the many named choices are:

1. Six Sigma (Define, Measure, Analyze, Improve, Control or DMAIC)
2. Lean, "Toyota"
3. Plan, Do, Check, Act (PDCA Cycle)
4. Theory of Constraints
5. Just in Time
6. Total Quality Management/Continuous Quality Improvement

In general, most methodologies are somewhat similar. Where they may differ is in their particular focus and toolkit. For example, Lean encourages primary focus on eliminating waste, whereas Six Sigma encourages statistical analysis of processes. It does not matter if you follow a specific approach or blend a combination of methods. What is important is that you adopt a standard approach, incorporate some degree of statistical analysis to model the behavior or actions of the process, and then develop consensus around potential improvements. A general process improvement methodology is shown in Figure 4-4.

Developing New Projects

Once the new PI department gains maturity, management should shift its focus toward developing a portfolio of projects. This is done by working with customers to identify and create a demand for services. Case studies of successes in initial projects are always helpful in encouraging other departments to visualize the results the department is capable of obtaining.

A request form is sometimes used by ME departments to obtain needed resources, with common elements of the form including the project's scope, background and business drivers, as well as timelines and deadlines. The project intake process, defined next, is essential to ensuring that the project is achievable and helps to increase value.

Measuring Project Status

The portfolio of projects that are currently underway in large ME groups can often be counted in the dozens. Even small groups will have a handful. Understanding and communicating the current status and overall risk with managers, customers and other stakeholders can be difficult. Groups should adopt some form of dashboard to allow quick visualization of status and alert the reader of the report to any potential problems.

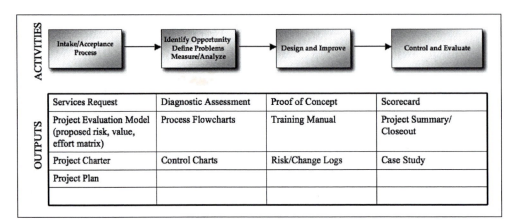

ACTIVITIES	Intake/Acceptance Process	Identify Opportunity Define Problems Measure/Analyze	Design and Improve	Control and Evaluate

OUTPUTS	Services Request	Diagnostic Assessment	Proof of Concept	Scorecard
	Project Evaluation Model (proposed risk, value, effort matrix)	Process Flowcharts	Training Manual	Project Summary/ Closeout
	Project Charter	Control Charts	Risk/Change Logs	Case Study
	Project Plan			

Figure 4-4: Process Improvement Methodology

Project Name	Analyst	% Work Complete / Total Effort	Next Major Milestone	Schedule/ Budget	Risk
Clinical EMR Rollout to first 2 units	Smith	95% / 600 days	Seeking CNO approval in May	Green	Green
Financial record automation process	Bobbins	72% / 320 days	Mid-February final rollout to all users; Resolve data exceptions	Red	Green
Implementation of patient portals	Craft	25% / 3 months	Finalize manuals, customer reports, and fix critical bugs. Update sponsor this week	Yellow	Red
Modeling and queuing project for emergency department	Roosevelt	70% / 4 months	Presented findings to Dr. Cox; mtg with sr. level management	Green	Green
Supply chain streamlining	Moore	3% / On Hold	Pending upgrades to forecasting system; Value Streams finalized	Yellow	Yellow

Figure 4-5: Project Portfolio Dashboard

One commonly used method to achieve this is through a frequently updated scorecard, or dashboard, which tracks progress and identifies key aspects of the project. A sample dashboard, using a "stoplight" approach, is shown in Figure 4-5.

EVALUATING POTENTIAL PROJECTS: PROJECT INTAKE

One of the critical steps in managing a process improvement function is to closely examine how projects are selected. Given constraints in financial and human resources, as all organizations have, it is critical to have a project intake, or acceptance process that selects projects which are of high strategic value and which optimize given resources.

Management engineering projects tend to encompass multiple functions, disciplines and operational areas within a hospital. In this respect, MEs often face challenges of supporting multiple end-user groups, each with conflicting objectives and resource needs. Proper allocation of resources should be done by considering three key factors: (1) financial impact (F) related to economic value generated by the organization; (2) productivity impact and operational performance (P) involving effect on human and physical resources; and (3) strategic alignment (A), measured by how well a project complies with the hospital's strategy. These dimensions (abbreviated here as FPA), summarize the relevant business drivers and provide a framework for the justification, implementation and long-term evaluation of new initiatives. Ideally, an organization selects a project that rates high in FPA dimensions, which makes it more likely that it will help maximize outcomes. Understanding how to incorporate the concept of FPA into a project development process, however, can be challenging and frustrating. Here we will present a framework to be used in the delivery and assessment of effective ME projects.

The ultimate result is to present an objective approach to review and justify a project proposal. We start by reexamining the NPV approach for selection of a project, followed by other approaches to valuing a project's impact in the organization.

Comparing Financial Impact: Net Present Value

An information technology project, like any other investment, does not have guaranteed returns or payoffs. Several levels of returns, or even losses, may take place in the future, and this uncertainty is what defines a project's risk level. As payoffs vary by project, however, how is it possible to compare different projects? A common approach is through the use of NPV, which, as seen in the following formula, discounts a project's present and future costs and benefits by using the project's risk level as a component of the discount factor.

$$NPV_i = \Sigma^t \, (B_t - C_t) \, / \, (1 - r)^t$$

The *r* in the formula is the risk level specific to the project. Several factors, such as demand for the products and technology, determine the level of risk involved with a specific project; however, at the institutional level, the following criteria can be used to define a project's risk level:

- Length of time required to implement the project
- Existing skills and experience implementing similar projects
- Technical complexity involved in the implementation
- End-user and management level of support for the project
- Magnitude of the change brought about with the project

Taking into account all of these factors and summarizing them into a single measurement of risk is extremely difficult. A practical approach is to make a subjective assessment involving a group of individuals not involved in the project. The group is asked to assign projects, based on the specified criteria, into one of three categories: low risk, medium risk and high risk. Once the projects have been assigned, the NPV can be calculated for each project, using the ranges of *r* levels as shown in Table 4-1.

Table 4-1: Risk Levels

Risk level	*r* range
Low	< 5%
Medium	5% to 10%
High	> 10%

Table 4-2 shows an example of two project's cash flows, with varying levels of risk.

Although depending on the useful project life, the analysis is normally done considering a five-year period. Rather than obtaining a single value for NPV, it is preferable to provide a range of NPV values, which allows managers more room for decision making, as Table 4-3 shows. In this case, Project 1 appears to be less attractive than Project 2. If both projects are considered low risk, Project 1 would be preferred over Project 2. However, if both projects are considered medium risk, then Project 2

Table 4-2: Project Comparison

		FY1	FY2	FY3	FY4	FY5	Total
Project 1	Expected Revenue Costs	$290,000	$50,000	$75,000	$100,000	$150,000	
	Benefits	($290,000)	$50,000	$75,000	$100,000	$150,000	$85,000
Project 2	Expected Revenue Costs	$290,000	$150,000	$125,000	$50,000	$25,000	
	Benefits	($290,000)	$150,000	$125,000	$50,000	$25,000	$60,000

Table 4-3: Project Comparison with Risk Analyses

		Low Risk		Medium Risk		High Risk	
Project 1	Risk rate	3%	5%	6%	10%	11%	15%
	Discounted factor (1+r)	1.03	1.05	1.06	1.10	1.11	1.15
	Net present value	$52,452	$33,748	$25,184	($4,526)	($10,950)	($33,301)
Project 2	Risk rate	3%	5%	6%	10%	11%	15%
	Discounted factor (1+r)	1.03	1.05	1.06	1.10	1.11	1.15
	Net present value	$40,218	$28,567	$23,153	$3,919	($346)	($15,546)

would be preferable over Project 1. Finally, if both projects are considered high-risk, neither project should be implemented.

Measuring Expected Productivity Impact

One measurement that is rarely considered in project resource allocation is expected impact on productivity and human resources. A simple approach to decompose changes resulting from new technology is the use of ratio comparison, which has been used for analysis in cost changes[1] and expenditure analysis.[2]

Using the following model we can decompose changes in total production into changes in productivity or personnel:

$$\text{Change in Total Production} = I_2 * (P_2 - P_1) + P_1 * (I_2 - I_1)$$

Where I_i is the level of FTEs for period the ith and P_i is the level of productivity per FTE for the ith period.

Thus, in a case of two projects showing exactly the same level of potential production, as shown in Table 4-4, the cause of change can be different.

Table 4-4: Project Comparison with Production Changes

		Project 1	Project 2
Present	Current FTEs	10	15
	Current productivity per FTE	3	2
	Total production	30	30
Expected	Future FTEs	9	12
	Future productivity per FTE	4	3
	Total production	36	36
Total change due to productivity changes		9	12
Total change due to FTE changes		–3	–6
Total production change		2	6

Table 4-4 shows that Project 2 has the advantage of larger changes in production due to productivity improvements. However, this improvement comes as the result of large decreases in labor. If the objective of the institution is to reduce personnel, this project would be acceptable, but when there are concerns of reassigning employees (a condition common in not-for-profit hospitals), Project 1 would be more acceptable. Likewise, projects that impact large increments in productivity can be an objective, even at the sacrifice of FTEs. This latter approach can be implemented in cases for which opportunities to allocate displaced FTEs in high-value activities exist.

Evaluating a Project's Strategic Alignment

An assessment of a project's potential is not complete without an idea of how it meets the strategic goals of the organization. An approach to measuring strategic alignment uses a score or index. One concept along this line, which has been discussed, is using a system of four factors to determine the outcome of any transformation initiative; these factors are called DICE, or *duration, integrity, commitment,* and *effort*.[3] Based on scores for each area, it becomes possible to predict potential outcomes.

There are several components in establishing the score of a new project: (1) perceived alignment with institutional strategic goals and organizational outcomes; (2) support from senior management; and (3) acceptance on the part of end-users. We developed an approach to predicting impact for a project, using five total factors. As shown in Table 4-5, the score for each category can take a value ranging from 1 to 4, with the lowest value representing a high contribution to the success of the project and the highest value representing the least favorable conditions for success of the project. Applying the formula and using the weights assigned in the table, the best overall score for a project can be a 7, whereas the worst possible is 28.

Based on a scaling system such as this, it is possible to define the strategic importance of any project. For example, a project with a score of less than 14 would be considered of significant strategic importance to the institution, whereas those scoring 14 to 20 are less important from the institution's strategic point of view.

Table 4-5: Strategic Alignment Factors

Factors for Defining Project Strategic Alignment	Points (1–4)
Impact on organizational outcomes (e.g., market share, patient satisfaction) [X_1]	1
Potential for performance improvement [X_2]	2
Project integration: alignment with current projects [X_3]	1
Executive sponsorship and commitment [X_4]	2
Customer/end-user commitment [X_5]	2
Weighted score = $X_1 + (2^* X_2) + (2^* X_3) + X_4 + X_5 = 11$	

Providing a Final Score for the Project

The final assessments include the multi-factor description and ranking of the best projects. The overall result is a list of projects ordered in a queue, with the queue formed from consideration of the items previously described.

A summary of ranking for two illustrative cases is given in Table 4-6.

Table 4-6: Project Evaluation Summary

Evaluation Type	Project 1	Project 2
Financial/NPV	Medium	Low
Productivity impact	Low	High
Strategic alignment	Medium	High

Transforming each level into numeric values (Low=1, Medium=2 and High=3) gives us a comparative measure for the two projects. Ideally, where demand for multiple projects exists, organizations should choose one which maximizes all three areas. Figure 4-6 shows a "radar diagram" with three dimensions (financial, performance,

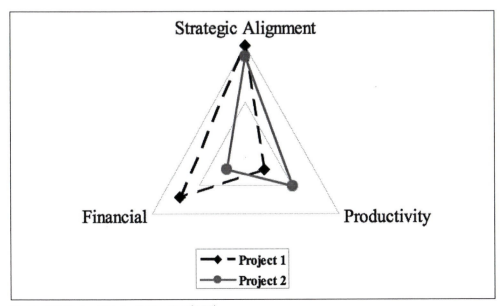

Figure 4-6: Project Intake Evaluation (APF)

and alignment) and a comparison of two projects, in which Project 1 ranks higher on strategic alignment and financial outcomes, and Project 2 is stronger on productivity impacts. Based on this summary diagram, Project 1 would appear to maximize all the three dimensions.

Six Sigma and Process Modeling

Once projects have been selected and teams assigned, the first step in all methodologies is to understand the behavior of the processes under review. Building this understanding starts by comprehensively modeling the process, activity by activity. The process of modeling should attempt to define each of these:

- **Activity:** A task which occurs at a specific point in time, has a duration that is random and shows a known probability distribution function.
- **Time:** A key parameter of a process, defined as the differential between the time an activity started and ended.
- **Event:** The culmination of an activity, which can change the state of a process.
- **Outcomes:** The results of the activities and events, most commonly expressed in a metric to gauge success and failure.

Most methodologies attempt to model each activity and event by carefully observing and documenting the components just defined. For example, if a nurse enters a room to take vital signs at 10:05 a.m. and leaves at 10:22 a.m. with three procedures completed, the output matrix would look like what is shown in Table 4-7.

Table 4-7: Process Model

Activity	Time	Event	Outcome
Nurse intervention	17 min., 0 sec.	Nurse completes 3 procedures	Successful

After adequate observation of these activities, which normally involves a significant period of time, the process can be modeled, using traditional process flowchart tools. More importantly, the *behavior* of the activities can be statistically analyzed, which is one of the main contributions of the Six Sigma methodology. Some may argue that Six Sigma has no role in medicine; we disagree and believe that all processes can benefit from a better understanding of behaviors.

Modeling the time intervals allows engineers to understand the variability of the process. **Variability** is the range of possible outcomes of a given process. It is also defined as the amount of dispersion around the mean, or the inconsistency of results. The greater the variability, the less control exists in the process outcomes. Both standard deviations and variance are the primary statistical measures of variability, although standard deviation is probably more widely used and definitely applied in Six Sigma. In a normally distributed set of data, +/– one standard deviation from the mean will include 68.2% of all observations, and two standard deviations represent 95% of all observations. The mean is typically represented by the Greek symbol (x) and standard deviation by the Greek symbol sigma (σ), defined as the square root of the variance.

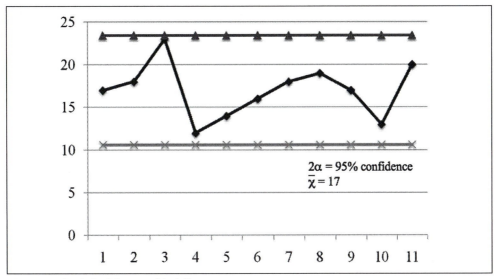

Figure 4-7: Statistical Process Modeling

For example, assume we have 11 observations of nursing data, ranging from 11 to 23 minutes. The mean is approximately 17, and the standard deviation of these data is 3.193. Therefore, within 1σ deviation from the mean would be approximately 20.2 and 2σ (or the 95% confidence interval) would be 23.4 minutes. Therefore, in 68% of the cases, nurses were likely to complete their three procedures between 13.8 and 20.2 minutes. In 95% of the cases, you could expect that nurses would complete their three procedures in no more than 23.4 minutes and no less than 10.6 minutes. Understanding the behavior of data at a statistical level allows engineers to truly understand expectations and map out realistic process models. Figure 4-7 shows these concepts graphically.

Defect per Million Opportunities

Using process models and Six Sigma, engineers can capture several additional constructs. The first is the idea of an outcome known as a "defect." A **defect** is any instance in a process at which the customer requirement has not been met. In the earlier example of nursing procedures, the outcome was positive (i.e., they were successfully completed in 17 minutes). If however, it took 22 minutes for the procedures, and the patient was not able to have one of the three procedures completed, it would have been recorded as a defect, since it deviated from the expectation and did not meet the customer (or patient's) expectations. Six Sigma uses a metric known as Defect per Million Opportunities, or DPMO, to understand defect behavior for activities and processes.

To calculate DPMO, simply follow four steps:

- **Step 1:** Identify the process to evaluate and the specific deliverables produced by the process. In our nursing example, the process is nursing procedures and the deliverables are successful completion of three procedures.
- **Step 2:** Define successful outcomes and defects, and count the total number of opportunities. In our example, we defined the defect earlier. The total opportunities would be defined as: # of patients $\times$ # of procedures $\times$ frequency.

For example, if we had 20 patients, each requiring three procedures twice a day, the total number of opportunities would be 120 (or 20 × 3 × 2).

- **Step 3:** Obtain a statistical model of the process. In this step, the engineer should observe all the activities, gather the outcomes (as shown earlier), and statistically model the results, calculating the mean, standard deviation and control limits. In addition, the total number of defects should be counted and recorded. For example, if the engineer observed all 120 opportunities in one day and counted 8 defects (or instances that did not conform to requirements), then the DPMO would be calculated as: (8 ÷ 120) × 1,000,000 = 66,667. Therefore, in this example, the defects per million opportunities would be 66,667 (.06667 × 10^6).

- **Step 4:** Measure Sigma Level and manage improvements. After the DPMO is calculated, it is compared with a Six Sigma Level to obtain a measure of improvement opportunities. Six Sigma actually refers to the calculation in which only 3.4 defects per million is recorded, which yields a 99.99966% success rate. This yield can be calculated by subtracting from 100% the defect rate (e.g., 100% – (3.4/1,000,000) = 100 – .00034 = .99966, or 99.9%. Figure 4-8 allows you to graphically compare your process's defect rates against Sigma and DPMO levels. Using the example from earlier (with more than 66,000 DPMOs), this would be Sigma level 3.

Process Capability Index

One other useful analytical tool that Six Sigma has provided is the process capability index (often expressed as C_p). A **process capability index** is a measure for gauging

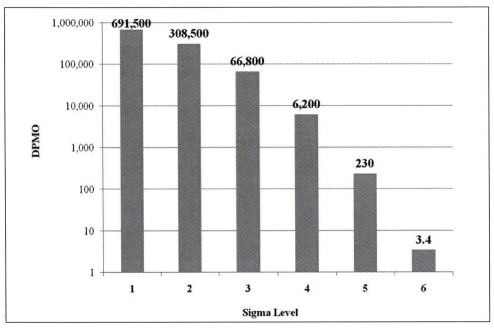

Figure 4-8: Six Sigma Levels and DPMO

the extent to which a process meets the customer's expectations. It is mathematically defined as:

[(Upper Standard Limit – Lower Standard Limit) ÷ 6σ]

A C_p > 1 suggests that the process is capable, but it does not have any relation to the performance target, nor does it suggest that the process meets the customers' expectations. To improve on this, other complimentary metrics should be used (such as C_{pk}). C_{pk} is defined as the minimum of either C_{pu} [(USL – x) ÷ 3σ] or C_{pl} [(x – LSL) ÷ 3σ].

RECOMMENDATIONS

To gain positive initial momentum, it is important to start off by selecting the right projects and focusing on creating value. There are several recommendations for ensuring that your new PI department is successful.

New Departments Take Time

It is a natural expectation that consultants hope for immediate results, but in complex organizations, even PI departments take time to cultivate. New initiatives tend to be seen as disruptions to the status quo or to people's areas of comfort, and resistance to change almost always exists. We recommend setting an expectation for a new department that allows it to start slowly—helping to address projects systematically and developing necessary tools, documentation and methodology precisely and with rigor.

Train Your PI Professionals

Do not allow PI analysts to work on a project if they are not prepared or trained. However, there is not a comprehensive training program that can help you educate your PI or MEs. This is often a critical bottleneck as new departments roll out, and a sure way for a project to fail is to staff it with an engineer who does not understand the methodologies or tools or lacks facilitation or project management skills. If this happens in the early stages, the fate of the new department is questionable at best. The initial results will dictate how successful the group will be in the long term, since it is nearly impossible to reverse the early perceptions of clients and management.

Experience, education, former project experience, and former healthcare training are all important, but they do not really help to teach your employee how to become a better analyst or project professional in PI. Although some associations and groups (such as HIMSS' Management Engineering-Performance Improvement Task Force) offer educational webinars and tools, you will likely have to develop a custom educational program using a variety of Web sites, conferences, books and societies to really jump start a good PI department.

Avoid Getting Mired in Bureaucracy

Large organizations have divisions with multiple departments that have a focus that is similar to PI or ME. It is important to view these departments as partners, helping to collaboratively achieve results, and not as competitors. Internal competition not only directs your efforts in the wrong direction, it distracts you from getting critical successes early in the department's development, educating your staff and formalizing your methodologies. These are the critical tasks that must remain the focus of management.

Focus on Initial Success and Creating Value

One of the things that successful PI departments do is to keep focused on business value, whether it is measured in better clinical quality, cycle-time reductions, cost improvements, enhanced internal controls or any other measurements. Focus on the real objective of ME or PI—improving business performance—needs to always be on the top of the list in the early years of formation.

To do this, projects need to have formal closure by preparation of a rigorous case study or post-project review that essentially documents the change in process and outcomes as a result of the initiative. These reviews should explore the gaps between initial and final performance indicators of the project. Converting these metrics into a value will allow management to share results and gain momentum.

This success, or value, increases the demand for services in the future. The amount of demand for project or PI work is one measure of how well the department is doing internally.

SUMMARY

Managing the PI function is extremely complex. While other functions eventually become routine and operationalized, the job of an ME or performance analyst is to constantly be immersed in something new—a new process, a new system, new customers, new departments and new locations. Understanding the basics of project management structure, which can be adapted and applied in many ways over time, is essential to repeated success. Developing a department or unit to perform PI requires leadership, hiring the right people, adopting good methods, selecting the right projects and managing for results. The use of Six Sigma tools and methods, especially statistical process control to analyze process behavior and measurement of defects and process capabilities, represents a great opportunity for healthcare process improvement. Management of all these areas is vital to performance improvement success.

References

1. Peden EA, Lee ML. Output and inflation components of medical care and other spending changes. *Healthcare Financing Review.* 1991; 13:75.
2. Huber M. Health expenditure trends in OECD countries, 1970-1997. *Healthcare Financing Review.* 1999; 21:99.
3. Sirkin HL, Keenan P, Jackson A. The hard side of change management. *Harvard Business Review.* 2005; October:109-118.

CHAPTER 5

Projects and Change

Rigoberto Delgado and James Langabeer II

> *"He who rejects change is the architect of decay. The only human institution which rejects progress is the cemetery."*
> — Harold Wilson, former U.K. Prime Minister

INTRODUCTION

Projects are undertaken to create value and improve performance. A **project** is defined here as an organized effort involving a sequence of activities that are temporarily performed to achieve a desired outcome. Being temporary and involving a variety of individuals and activities, it is important that projects be appropriately organized and managed. Similarly, the change that results from projects also must be closely managed. This chapter will discuss how PI professionals can use project management methods and tools to maximize benefits and minimize the disruptions that change creates.

THE BASICS OF PROJECT MANAGEMENT

The desired outcome for a project is typically defined as a combination of being on-time, on-budget, and on-scope. The previous chapter discussed ways in which projects must be aligned to produce real value, being aligned with strategic goals, having desirable productivity or performance impacts and creating economic value. All of these outcomes are achievable, but the ME plays a big role in ensuring the deliverables are met.

Projects move through multiple phases, from initial business case justification to project design, analysis, implementation and post-project reviews. This was shown in Figure 4-4 in Chapter 4. Once the project has been initiated, it is of the utmost importance to immediately provide control, or management to ensure that the project progresses as planned to avoid surprises and delays. This is the planning aspect of project management.

Planning Projects

In many large projects, especially information systems implementations, there might be thousands of activities (or tasks) to be performed by dozens of people (or resources).

	Name	Duration	Start	Predecessors	Resource names	December / Dec	January / Jan	February / Feb	March / Mar	April / Apr
1	⊞ Scope	3.5 d	01/03/00							
7	⊞ Analysis/S Scope Requirements	14 d	01/06/00							
17	⊟ Design	14.5 d	01/26/00							
18	Review preliminary software specificati...	2 d	01/26/00	16	Analyst					
19	Develop functional specifications	5 d	01/28/00	18	Analyst					
20	Develop prototype based on functional ...	4 d	02/04/00	19	Analyst					
21	Review functional specifications	2 d	02/10/00	20	Management					
22	Incorporate feedback into functional sp...	1 d	02/14/00	21	Management					
23	Obtain approval to proceed	4 h	02/15/00	22	Management,Proje...					
24	Design complete	0 d	02/15/00	23						
25	⊟ Development	21.75 d	02/16/00							
26	Review functional specifications	1 d	02/16/00	24	Developer					
27	Identify modular/tiered design parameters	1 d	02/17/00	26	Developer					
28	Assign development staff	1 d	02/18/00	27	Developer					
29	Develop code	15 d	02/21/00	28	Developer					
30	Developer testing (primary debugging)	15 d	02/24/00	29	Developer					
31	Development complete	0 d	03/18/00	30						
32	⊞ Testing	48.75 d	02/16/00							
46	⊞ Training	45.75 d	02/16/00							
57	⊞ Documentation	30.5 d	02/16/00							
67	⊞ Pilot	70.25 d	01/26/00							
74	⊞ Deployment	5 d	05/03/00							
81	⊞ Post Implementation Review	3 d	05/10/00							
86	Software development template complete	0 d	05/15/00	85						

Figure 5-1: Sample Project Plan

To track these activities and resources over time, while predicting and monitoring progress, it is necessary to use several tracking mechanisms. A Gantt chart is typically used as the project plan in large projects. Figure 5-1 shows a visual graphic of a project plan or Gantt chart.

Analytical methods such as program evaluation and review technique (PERT) and critical path method (CPM) are very similar ways of estimating the most desirable path to achieving the deliverables (on-time and within budget). Both methods attempt to arrange the project plan activities in such a way as to minimize total times by identifying the longest (or most critical) path and building the tasks around it. Program evaluation and review technique uses a simple formula that combines the most optimistic, or best-case times (O); most pessimistic, or worst-case times (P); and most likely expected times (M). The formula is expressed as the sum of the optimistic (O) and pessimistic (P) times, plus 4 times the most likely (M), the total of which is divided by 6. Mathematically, this is expressed as:

$$PERT = [O + P + 4M] \div 6$$

If a project is most likely to require 10 working days, in the worst case could actually require 20 days, but could in ideal circumstances be completed in 5 days, then PERT would suggest that the engineer should use 10.83 days as the expected project duration. This is a very valuable technique for estimating projects, but must be based on thorough examination of all details in the project plan.

In most cases, the project's start date is assigned based on funding or approval timing. The end-date, or project completion date, is usually determined in one of three ways:

1. Sometimes it is "mandated," as an executive order, legal or regulatory timeline, or other constraints.

2. Sometimes it is computed mathematically through a bottom-up approach, using PERT or CPM to add up all project tasks and realistically determine timelines.

3. Using a top-down "rough cut" planning process, key activities are discussed and critical paths are explored for these high-level events.

Once a project has defined the start and end dates, the project plan is essentially one of breaking tasks into specific functions by each responsible party. This is sometimes referred to as *work breakdown structure*, or WBS.

When planning projects, it is advisable to use a "charter" document, which describes the project charter, plans, assumptions and roles. This document helps to lay the foundation for how a project will be organized. An example is provided in Figure 5-2.

Organizing Projects

As project planning involves dividing up tasks by role, it is usually necessary to include a project organization chart that clarifies roles, responsibilities and parties involved in the process dedicated to the specific project. This includes clear delineation of the sponsor, project manager, functional leads, and staff support roles for each project. Figure 5-3 shows a sample project organization chart for this project.

Since projects typically are ad hoc and temporary, they most often involve matrix organizational structures in which daily operational reporting roles are clearly delineated or superimposed by the project structure. Such matrix organizations are very common in healthcare projects today.

Controlling Projects

When projects are begun, clear communication with all project members must be initiated to set ground rules for behavior and expectations. These expectations can be defined formally, in service level agreements between the project manager and the individual (see for example, Chapter 12 on service level agreement [SLA] structures) or they can be generic for the entire team. These expectations include:

- Understanding of attendance expectations and frequency of project meetings
- Expectations for getting things done intra-meeting
- Commitment levels, both in team meetings and as members are back in their operational roles
- Confidentiality
- Openness and candor during brainstorming sessions
- Roles in projects, such as meeting timekeeper, facilitator, recorder, parking lot attendant for notes and ideas, and other roles
- How to deal with conflict resolution

Keeping the project team focused on outcomes and progress is one way to ensure that teams do not become mired in bureaucracy or focused on negative tasks. Focus is ensured by reviewing project dashboards and focusing on strategic project frameworks. A strategic project framework is a simple, one-page summary of the key project objectives, activities, metrics and goals. A sample framework for one project, conducted for a large hospital supply chain and materials management department, is shown in Figure 5-4.

Project Charter Form (Sample)

Project Name:

Division:

Product/Process:

Prepared by:

Version Control:

PROJECT CHARTER PURPOSE
<Describe the high level charter or purpose of the project.>

PROJECT EXECUTIVE SUMMARY
<Summarize the key points of each of the following: Business requirements, scope, goals, objectives, estimates, work plan, budget, and overall approach.>

PROJECT JUSTIFICATION
<Briefly describe the rationale and business justification for undertaking this project.>

PROJECT SCOPE

Goals and Objectives

Goals	Objectives
1.	
2.	

Organizational Impacts

Organization	Estimated Impact

Project Deliverables

Milestone	Deliverable
1. <Milestone Description>	• <Deliverable 1—description> • <Deliverable 2—description> • <Deliverable n—description>
2. <Milestone Description>	• <Deliverable 1—description> • <Deliverable 2—description>

Deliverables Out of Scope
<List anything that is out of scope or that the project will explicitly consider.>

Project Estimated Costs & Duration

Project Key Milestone	Date Estimate	Deliverable(s) Included	Confidence Level
<Milestone 1>		<Deliverable 1> <Deliverable 2>	<High/Medium/Low>
<Milestone 2>		<Deliverable 1>	<High/Medium/Low>

Figure 5-2: Sample Project Charter Form

PROJECT CRITERIA

Project Assumptions
- <Assumption 1>
- <Assumption 2>
- <Assumption 3>

Forecasted Project Issues

Priority Criteria

High-priority issue impacting critical path. Immediate resolution required.

Medium-priority issue, requiring mitigation before next milestone.

Low-priority issue, and can be resolved prior to project completion.

#	Date	Priority	Owner	Description	Status & Resolution
1				<Issue 1 description>	<Resolution>
2				<Issue 2 description>	<Resolution>

Forecasted Project Risks

#	Risk Area	Likelihood	Risk Owner	Project Impact-Mitigation Plan
1	<Project Risk>	H, M, L		<Mitigation Plan>
2				

Project Constraints
- <Constraint 1>
- <Constraint 2>

Project Team Organization Plans

Project Team Role	Project Team Member(s)	Responsibilities
<Role, Title>		

APPROVALS

_____   _____

Project Manager   Executive Sponsor

Figure 5-2: Sample Project Charter Form *(continued)*

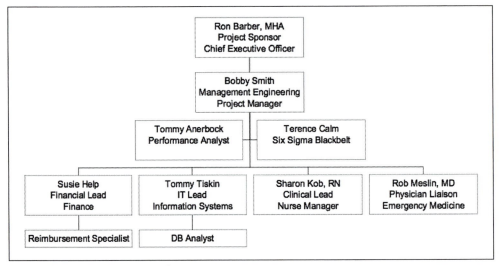

Figure 5-3: Project Organization Chart

Project Objectives	*Become Seamless*	*Automate Processes*	*Become Financially Effective*	*Retain and Recruit Talent*
Operational Activities	•Attend Nursing and clinical meetings •Create service level agreements with customers •Partner with vendors •Update Policy and Procedures manual •Forecasting Inventory	•Warehouse scanning solution •Business intelligence reporting	•Establish consignment inventory programs when possible	•Identify current skill sets of employees •Determine skill sets necessary for future roles •Include employee input on policies and procedures
Key Performance Indicators	•Improved communication with customers •Reduced inventory risk •Improved vendor relationships •Improved efficiencies •Reduced stock-outs	•Improved productivity •Better reporting to analyze costs, improve compliance, and drive standardization	•Improved inventory utilization •Reduced days inventory on hand	•Implement quarterly employee survey •Reduced loss of personnel to other departments
Goals	•Reduction in complaints >10% •Reduction in stock outs by 20%	•Decreased data entry time for requisitions >10% •Reduction in data entry errors >10%	•Inventory value for both warehouses =<$500,000 •Decreased days inventory on hand > 5 days	•Ensure each employee receives 24 hours training per year

Figure 5-4: Strategic Project Framework

CHANGE

Process improvement efforts result in change, which occurs to both individuals and the organization as a whole. Though change might be beneficial in the long run, in the near term it creates ambiguity, confusion and tension if not appropriately managed. During the *control* phase of the project, PI professionals need to develop a change management plan for each project to minimize disruptions and ensure that the improvements stabilize and remain over time. The overall purpose of the change plan is to implement ways of amplifying the project's driving forces and shrinking the resistance forces. The elements of each phase are outlined below.

Create the Conditions for Change

The first step in creating the conditions for change is to communicate the gap between the current state and the end state. This requires securing buy-in from sponsors and support from the top. This is an important component of the communication strategy as it relates the key players in the change process. Communicate change to all those affected, identify potential opposition and contact potential sponsors.

Next, it is important to create a sense of urgency. This is accomplished by presenting demonstrations on new technology, emphasizing the benefits of making the change, such as shorter cycle, paperless, higher security and efficiency.

Finally, all must agree on a change plan and timeline for achieving the end state. At the end of the testing cycle, the ME or project manager will conduct an evaluation of deliverables and will secure approval from management to proceed with full-scale deployment of the project.

Make Change Happen

The following four key activities cause change to occur:

1. Developing awareness, communication and training programs tailored to each target group. All of the users who will be impacted, as well other stakeholders, need to be prepared in advance for the changes that will occur.
2. Creating and communicating the vision. This is a critical element in guiding the change effort. The key factor, however, is to provide an actionable mission, a concise statement that articulates the purpose of the new process, system or solution. For example, a vision for a new patient kiosk in a clinic might be to "make patient registration fast and easy."
3. Forming an advisory or empowerment team. The team will consist of no more than four advisors representing different user segments. Regular meetings with the advisory team should improve communication, help identify and eliminate bottlenecks and determine how to handle resistance.
4. Publicizing the transformation target date. This is the date when the new process will replace an existing process. Understanding timelines and dates helps impacted users understand the changes to come.

Make Change Stick

Once you have created the conditions for change and successfully made the change, it becomes important that it remain in place when members of the project team disband and return to their original positions. This is not as easy as one might expect.[1]

One of the first guidelines for making change stick is to maintain the empowering structures for a period of time post-project. The objective is to open channels of communication with the end-user community. Retaining the advisory team for six months after the new process or solution go-live date is a good idea. If a help desk is used for the transition (for instance in the case of a large system migration or implementation), it could be used to analyze call patterns and periodically make proactive calls to users to ensure usage and understanding of the new solution. If comment or suggestion boxes are used, they can help to gather ideas and to keep the user community involved and active in the process.

It is also necessary to identify and minimize barriers to change. Removing structures that hinder the optimal functioning of the new process is a critical step in the success of the project. Identifying barriers will result from the work of the advisory team and using feedback from the help desk. Removing those barriers, however, will involve interactions with management.

Organizations also might consider implementing financial incentives. Individuals involved in implementing new projects should receive financial rewards based on the goals of the project and clear KPI objectives.

Lastly, making change stick involves measuring and communicating the value (e.g., economic, cycle time, patient satisfaction) gained with the new process or system. The impact assessment is the final phase of the project management process, and its goal is to provide management with objective data on the benefits of the new solution and to gain support for follow-up projects. The results of the assessment should be shared with end-users to improve acceptance and encourage further improvement.

Roles in the Change Process

Developing a list of individuals to carry out the tasks of communication and promotion allows project managers to increase the potential for success. There are four broad roles:

1. Sponsors—People who legitimize and authorize the change
2. Change agents—Individuals who are tasked with planning and executing the change
3. Advocates—Those who request and support the change
4. Targets—Individuals who will have to live with the change, such as end-users

Each of these types has a role to play in the change process and ultimately helps to determine project outcomes.

PROJECT COMMUNICATION

Communication is vital to managing change.[2] Two components of communication plans are strategy and brand positioning. The strategy outlines the channels of communication, whereas the brand position statements define the message (content and direction).

Given its level of use among the target groups, e-mail is nearly always an important component of the communication strategy. Communication frequency needs to be outlined as well; the greater the change, the greater the need for more frequent communication. A strategy may include other elements as shown in Table 5-1.

In addition to detailing plans for communication strategy, brand positioning also needs to be outlined. This includes identification of the following two aspects.

Customer Need and Benefits

State what customer need or benefit to the user group will occur as a result of the project. If the process has a definite impact on the users, this should be amplified in all communication prior to the new process go-live. Time savings, elimination of manual entry, and reduction in rework, are all great benefits for customers. Brand positioning

Table 5-1: Communication Channels

Channel	Suggested Frequency (example)	Action
Mass-e-mail	Product release	Targeted mass mail-out
Employee forums	As needed	Article describing new process or solution
Newsletter	Quarterly	Article describing new solution
New employee orientation	As needed	Materials for the orientation packet

statements in communication should reinforce this list of benefits. An example is: "The new process will eliminate the need for you to make three copies of all invoices."

Brand Character

The communication style that is chosen should reflect the character of the new process or solution. For example, if a new automated system for patient registration is implemented, such as a self-service kiosk, the communication might use terms such as "effective," "painless," and "secure." Words play a very important part of the mindset and perception that will ultimately become reality.

PROJECT RISKS

Risks are positively correlated with the need for strong project management: the greater the potential risks, the greater the need for skilled facilitation, control and management. Risks may take many forms. One major risk is long project times. As projects stretch out into multiple quarters and years, they are more likely to encounter staff turnover, funding or other resource shifting and lower degrees of focus and momentum in later periods. Projects having a larger scale and scope also bring higher risks. Implementation of large numbers of electronic medical records in multiple hospitals, for example, involve wide scale and scope and are always complex. Cross-functional, multi-departmental projects are also high risk, as they may lose momentum or focus as they stretch boundaries. Other common risks, having to do with planning, fallibilities or organizational traits include lack of training, poor communication, lack of funding, organizational politics, and inadequate preparation on the part of the engineer or analyst. All of these can be avoided with careful risk management.

Many PI analysts worry more about potential risks than about the details of ensuring that deliverables and positive outcomes are generated. Although we disagree with this strategy, we believe it is important to identify and mitigate risks whenever possible. At a minimum, this entails documenting risks as they are discovered, logging them into the project database or files, sharing them with the project team and sponsors and identifying contingency plans in the event the risk materializes.

Figure 5-5 shows a summary of a risk issues log used in successful PI projects.

PROJECT MANAGEMENT OFFICE

In certain instances, MEs have helped to create a project management office. A **project management office** (PMO) is a group of professionals that assist management in

RISK MANAGEMENT LOG

Project: Emergency Department Capacity Analysis (Queuing Model)		Date: May 1, 2009	
Analyst: Moore			
Date Risk Identified	Risk Type	Risk Comments/Estimated Impact	Severity
07/05/08	Financial	Budget reduced by $500,000	Low
09/01/08	Personnel	Lopez was re-assigned out of project, could delay project 6 weeks	High
01/04/09	Scope	Sponsor added three new goals	Low
03/01/09	Technical	Integration with ERP is poorly defined	Medium
05/01/09	Organizational	Merger underway with new system; could impact sustainability of project	Uncertain

Figure 5-5: Risk Issues Log

developing structure and standards for more sophisticated management of projects.[3] Typically, PMOs are created to assist in deployment of information technology and usually report to the chief information officer, although in reality, PMOs can be used for any type of organizational project. Since most large systems literally have dozens of large projects and hundreds of smaller IT projects in the portfolio, a PMO functions as the portfolio manager to some degree—ensuring that risks are being mitigated and that a comprehensive view of all projects is available for the CIO and other executives involved in the governance process.

The PMO has two primary roles:

1. Developing standards for governance (evaluation, planning, management and control) of projects, and ensuring that these standards are consistently followed across the organization.
2. Managing the organizational perspective of information technology, which primarily involves institutional project portfolio management.

Portfolio management is a widely used term in IT more recently but was actually "borrowed" from the financial sector where financial portfolios are commonly used. Although it has many definitions, portfolio management is defined here as "the systematic governance of projects with an aim toward maximizing value or utility across the organization, while managing risks."

With its focus on value creation, a PMO has to take the lead in ensuring that all projects have defined performance expectations (i.e., benefits are clearly documented in the project evaluation stages, and then on an ongoing basis both during the project and postimplementation). As many benefits are often described ambiguously (many times on purpose by project managers), PMOs have to consistently require and enforce quantitative expressions of benefits whenever possible as part of the governance processes. Management of the portfolio requires having a complete perspective on performance contributions per project.

Because of their skill sets, MEs and PI analysts are often selected to staff, consult or lead in PMO creation and management. Their expertise in metrics and methods helps ensure that the standards that are set are realistic and routinely applied to all projects. Development of accurate performance metrics is one of the biggest areas of opportunity.

Project management offices should be evaluated by their reach across the organization and for their project success rates defined as the percentage of projects that both (a) reach the desired milestones on-time, within budget and scope; and (b) achieve the deliverables (i.e., performance benefits) expressed in the governance process. To achieve this, PMOs need to develop a collaborative, consulting approach in which PMO analysts reach out to the organization and continuously offer advice and assistance. This might at times be in the form of tactical assistance in understanding documentation and methodologies, or as strategic assistance in resolving project issues and hitches. Given the focus of PMOs to help standardize processes, taking a "command and control" approach, in which mandates and a centralized approach to projects dominate, is destined to fail. PMOs should instead focus on developing a service-line approach. As such, PMOs services should offer:

- Training of project professionals throughout the organization
- Development and deployment of standards, methodologies and documentation
- Routine communication newsletters and updates to keep project managers engaged at a more strategic level
- Visibility on KPIs for key processes across the organization
- Evaluation, acquisition, and training around project software and tools

SUMMARY

Project management is a learned skill. Logically and efficiently organizing resources and activities produces more optimal results. Projects force change; however, and the principles and mechanisms for managing change should also be incorporated into projects. Communication strategies with brand positioning should be included on a regular basis in all communication with organizational stakeholders in order to prepare for changes. Risks should also be identified and mitigated.

References

1. Cameron E, Green M. *Making Sense of Change Management: A Complete Guide to the Models, Tools & Techniques of Organizational Change.* London: Kogan Page; 2004.
2. Englund RL, Graham, R, Dinsmore PC. *Creating the Project Office: A Manager's Guide to Leading Organizational Change.* San Francisco: John Wiley & Sons, Inc.; 2003.
3. Lewis JP. *Fundamentals of Project Management.* New York: AMACOM; 2006.

CHAPTER 6

Principles of Process Redesign

Kim Brant-Lucich

> *"Almost all quality improvement comes via simplification of design, manufacturing, layout, processes, and procedures."*
>
> — Tom Peters, management consultant

INTRODUCTION

The term *process improvement* is frequently used synonymously with performance improvement, process redesign and process reengineering. As with Shakespeare's rose, process improvement by any other name is still process improvement. A **process** is a set of steps that transform inputs into outputs, or activities performed in sequence to achieve a specific outcome. Merriam-Webster's dictionary, 11th edition, defines **improvement** as "something that enhances value or excellence." It follows, therefore, that a **process improvement** is anything that enhances the steps or activities of transforming an input into an output, or anything that makes the activities perform better (i.e., excellent). In the case of most processes, *better* would suggest greater efficiency and/or effectiveness— a more expedient process, fewer errors, minimal redundancy and reduced waste. Figure 6-1 is a high level, conceptual depiction of a process as something that is triggered by an event or action and which then transforms inputs into outputs. The text at the bottom of the figure provides an example of a sample process (i.e., medical office charting process).

As an acting teacher of mine always said, "It doesn't matter how you get there, as long as you get there." At a macro level, the same could be said of process improvement, though it would be naïve, and likely very costly, to assume that anything goes or that an approach or methodology is not required. The challenge is in determining what approach or methodology is right for your organization and what is right within the time, resource and cost constraints of the implementation. Approaches vary from simple process improvement driven by process modeling and analysis to technology-driven process simulation to Lean/Six Sigma. The point of my acting teacher's direction was to steer actors away from over-emphasizing method and toward results, which in the case of a process improvement, would be a process that is better than it was before

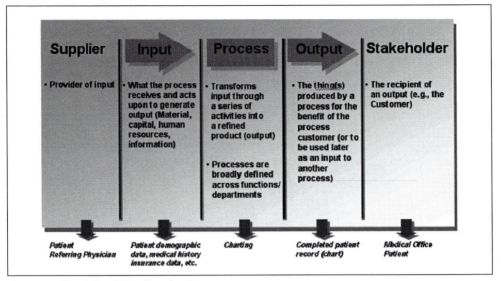

Figure 6-1: Physician Office Charting Process

the system implementation project began. Again, focusing on results, the same acting teacher used to say, "no one wants to see your homework."

As this translates to process improvement, it is usually the case that none involved, particularly executives, wants to see all of the process detail but prefer a high-level picture of challenges, improvement opportunities and results. Although management communications and reporting are worthy of a chapter of their own, suffice it to say that management communications should always be concise and to the point but inclusive enough to provide an accurate assessment of the situation.

The purpose of this chapter is to demystify the *art* of process improvement, purposely using the term *art* here because process improvement can be thought of more as an art rather than a science. Though it requires analysis and logic, a certain amount of creativity and intuition are necessary in its use. In addition, as people are involved in most processes, knowledge and understanding of human nature and organizational culture are also integral components of process improvement. This chapter will provide an overview of approaches to process improvement and will propose a very basic, reusable approach that can be integrated with system implementation to improve the likelihood of project success and user adoption.

THE IMPORTANCE OF PI IN SYSTEM IMPLEMENTATION

Numerous sources cite "failure to include process redesign" as one of the primary causes of system implementation failure, or failure of the implementation project to achieve its projected return on investment. In *CIO Insight*'s 2008 survey of the top priorities of CIOs, "improving business processes" was ranked as the second highest priority, right after "improving customer service."[1] Typically, an organization understands the need to include process analysis and change management as part of a system implementation. However, when budgets are being reviewed for project approval, the first thing to be eliminated is the line item that says "process analyst" or "change manager." When I worked as a consultant, I saw this repeatedly; clients balked at spending money on process improvement or change management. They merely wanted to "get the system in" as quickly and inexpensively as possible and did not consider as necessary the resources (people and time) required to analyze, document and improve processes as part of implementation.

The failure to invest in process improvement was so often the case that consultants disparagingly referred to it as "system slamming," or "slamming in the system" with no regard for the people or processes affected. Often, there is the assumption that processes can be revisited and refined once the system is in place. In fact, organizations view process work as unnecessary and often trade the individuals performing that function for those with the more technical skills of software development, interface development, testing, system training and project management. More often than not, the project manager is expected to manage change, which includes any changes to processes, policies and procedures. A good project manager may well have the ability to manage the system implementation life cycle as well as managing people, issues and risks, but if process improvement is not an integral and mandatory line item on a workplan, it is likely to be overlooked. Typically, a project manager might identify the need for process work, but the organization (or client) pushes back with the claim that there is not time for "a bunch of people to sit around doing process flows that will only end up in a notebook and never get looked at again."

The fact is that process flows often do end up in notebooks, which eventually become dusty. However, if a process is not assessed or improved prior to defining system requirements, then the requirements will be based on existing processes, and the system implementation will be nothing more than automation of the existing, and often poorly designed, process. The system, once implemented, may seem to add additional burdensome steps to the existing process, so users will find workarounds to avoid using the system and adoption will be low. When adoption is poor, there is little to no return on investment for the investment in information technology. It is generally at this point, which is after the fact, that organizations bring in a team to "fix" the implementation.

BASIC PROCESS IMPROVEMENT APPROACH

There are a variety of process improvement methodologies that can be applied to system implementation. Lean/Six Sigma has become the latest trend in the healthcare industry since about 2002, with numerous health organizations jumping on the band wagon, and a host of conferences and seminars dedicated to applying Toyota's Lean Production System to healthcare. However, prior to the push for Lean/Six Sigma, the standard approach was what I like to refer to as the "old fashioned method" of process improvement. This involves a few basic steps, which is not unlike the Lean approach:

1. Documentation and evaluation of existing processes (referred to as "current state" or "as is" process), and identification of risks and improvement opportunities
2. Visioning or design of the future state, or "to be" process
3. Gap analysis between the current and future state processes
4. Implementation plan for getting from the current state to the future state

To be truly comprehensive, all four of the steps should consider people, process and technology—people performing a process step, the process itself, and any enabling technology that supports (or does not support) the current or future state processes.

The gap analysis and implementation plans should address what needs to take place to bridge the gaps (e.g., communication and training, technology requirements, workflow redesign). These steps may seem like an oversimplification of the process but, in my experience, these are absolutely critical to beginning a process redesign effort and, more specifically, critical to system implementation. The four basic steps must be completed before process improvement can begin and before system development efforts start. Within those steps are varying degrees of rigor that may be applied, from root cause analysis to computerized process simulation, depending on the need, skill set of staff and availability of simulation tools.

Lean/Six Sigma

The Lean/Six Sigma approach to process improvement is similar in theory to the process described earlier, though the tools and methods differ, and a greater degree of rigor is applied to identifying and eliminating process waste (Lean) and reducing process variation (Six Sigma). Lean is a facilitative approach, engaging multiple users, documenting standard work, using process simulation (not computerized) to facilitate brainstorming of improvements and observing and timing processes. Statistical tools may also be applied, which is the point at which the "Six Sigma" component of Lean enters the picture. For an organization to use Lean as its standard approach to process improvement, Lean must be identified as an organizational strategy and must be embedded in the corporate culture. Using Lean requires strong senior leadership support and a well-trained staff with the skill sets required to facilitate Lean process improvement. It would be extremely naive to decide to use Lean/Six Sigma for one system implementation, if it is not the methodology currently in place across the enterprise. There are, however, many Lean tools which may be incorporated into "old fashioned process improvement," if team members are trained and skilled in the use of these tools. There are many books available on the subject of using Lean in healthcare, and I would urge anyone interested in using Lean for process improvement to do additional research. For the sake of viewing process improvement as it relates to system implementation, the rest of this chapter will focus on "old fashioned process improvement."

ASSESSING THE PROBLEM

Often, the request for a system implementation is driven by the emergence of new technologies, or it might be based on a regulatory mandate (for example, infection monitoring or electronic medical records). On the other hand, it may be requested to solve an identified problem. A hospital might determine that it needs an OR (operating room) scheduling application because of high physician dissatisfaction and time delays in its ORs. It is common to blame technology, or the lack of it, for such problems. However, it is spurious to assume, without analysis, that the problem will be solved with the implementation of a surgery scheduling application.

There might, in fact, be other inefficiencies. Until the process and root cause of the problem are appropriately identified and analyzed, it is premature to move toward a technical solution. For example, in the case of a request for a surgery scheduling application to better utilize the OR and manage patient flow, the issue causing the delays may be that the appropriate supplies are not on the surgical trays or carts when the doctor needs them. This problem could be the result of poor inventory management, or it might be that the physician's preferences have not been identified, or, as is often the case, it may be the result of poor workflow design or a complete absence of any documented standard workflow. These reasons cannot be uncovered until an objective third party evaluates the process and does some root cause analysis. Common approaches to root cause analysis are using a fishbone (Ishikawa) diagram or backing into the core problem by asking "why" repeatedly.

The problem is often not the first and most obvious identified process shortcoming. When an analyst drills down by asking "why" repeatedly, he or she should ultimately arrive at the root cause of the problem. Often, the root cause will be that there is no understood or documented process or procedure for part or all of a process. Sadly, it is uncommon for a process assessment to actually stop a system implementation from going forward. In most organizations, once a project has been selected, and there is momentum, it is rare for the plug to be pulled because a process analyst has determined that the intended system will not fix the problem. However, when the organization's project management structure contains procedures for risk management and issues management (which it should), it is quite reasonable for the analyst to identify this as a risk that project objectives will not be met. It is more likely that problems identified during the analytical process will merely identify opportunities for the system implementation team to build a system that will truly transform the existing processes, rather than merely automate them.

DOCUMENTING THE PROCESS

Evaluation and documentation of existing processes can be achieved through individual interviews, group process modeling sessions or process observation. The output of this exercise is, ideally, a process flow. Figure 6-2 is a process flow of a 'managed care member appeals process.' This process will be further described below.

The managed care member appeals process is the process by which a member of a managed care organization who has been denied care for any number of reasons, may challenge the managed care organization's decision. As part of a call center implementation at a managed care organization, this process was evaluated to identify the touch points and handoffs between the member, customer service representative, claims department and clinical review team. It was one of several processes evaluated as part of a call center implementation project. The objective of the system implementation was to service several different regions of the managed care organization with one centralized call center.

Prior to defining system requirements, it is critical to document existing processes and to identify process improvement opportunities that may or may not be enabled by the new technology. The primary reason for this is to ensure that the system will not be merely automating the existing process. Visual representation of the process is also useful for identifying risks and improvement opportunities and brainstorming future improvements. It can also be used as a schematic to show where systems interact with the process. This can be especially helpful when there are multiple systems that require interface development. Documenting the process supports identification of process improvements before system requirements are developed. Another valid reason for

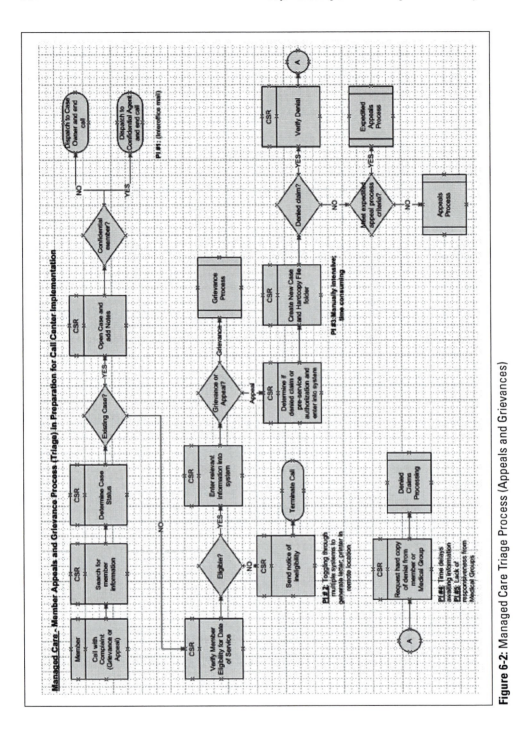

Figure 6-2: Managed Care Triage Process (Appeals and Grievances)

documenting the process with various stakeholders is to engage the future users up front in the design of their workflow as well as the system. As the future system users work through their existing process, they will not only identify improvement opportunities but will also begin to envision how the process might be enhanced, so that their contribution to the systems requirements development process will be invaluable.

The process flow should show who performs what activity. This can be done by labeling process boxes or by using a cross-functional process flow. Cross-functional flows are slightly more complex to create but are useful when a process crosses back and forth between multiple functional areas. Cross-functional flows also help identify lag times or present opportunities for processing that can be parallel, so that one functional area can continue to work fluidly, without being bound to wait for a hand-off from another process.

It is also useful, when documenting processes for the sake of system implementation, to create a matrix that identifies process triggers, inputs, outputs and metrics. Figure 6-3 includes information that should be captured as part of process assessment and incorporated into the system requirements definition process. Information can be gathered in single sheets per process or, more ideally, in an Excel or Word template or a business process modeling tool. There is a wealth of business process modeling tools available for this purpose, but be aware that some of these tools require significant staff training and, unless the tool has an easy-to-use process simulation module, may not be worth the time and money to get the process team up to speed on its use.

Collecting process detail may seem like a cumbersome activity, but it is important in the case of a system implementation to understand what triggers a process, all of the things that feed into the process (inputs) and the endpoint (outputs). It goes without saying that assumptions should always be captured because a faulty assumption can change everything about a process or about a system design. The knowledge required

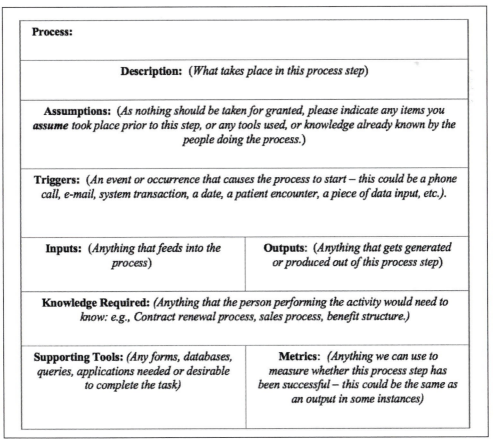

Figure 6-3: Key Process Components (Triggers, Inputs, Outputs, Metrics)

by staff or system users and the supporting tools are also important. These latter items feed into the training that will be developed.

Finally, metrics are a critical component as, assumedly, the purpose of the system implementation is to improve a particular process or the outcome of the process. It is necessary to determine a baseline metric (i.e., where the process is performing today), and to measure the result of the implementation against that baseline. It is often difficult to identify or compute a baseline, because a process might be very manual. It could require chart review or process observation to gain an understanding of current state baseline metrics. If a process is being observed, or charts are being reviewed, the reviewer should ensure that a random sample is observed or reviewed and that judgment is not being made based on anomalies. However metrics are identified, since the business case for a system implementation will no doubt include expected benefits, the starting point for those benefits (baseline) must be captured to understand whether the implementation has been a success.

Identifying and Engaging Stakeholders

Any system implementation in healthcare will have multiple stakeholders, ranging from the end customer, such as the patient, to the physicians, clinicians, unit secretaries, senior management, system users and others. Often, it may not be clear who all the stakeholders are until the process analysis begins. Typically, this is a top-down process, beginning with the project sponsor and ending with the end user of the process. The front-line workers who are closest to the process may be the best resource to help identify other impacted parties. In the process modeled earlier, the key stakeholder is the member who is appealing a health plan decision—either a denial of payment of a claim or a denial of future care (failure to pre-authorize care). Other process stakeholders are the member services representatives and physicians and clinicians involved in analyzing the appeal. Typically, the member services organization, claims organization, utilization review and clinical review may all reside in different areas of the organization.

I was involved in an implementation of this kind in which the entire process had been identified and documented, and system requirements definition and rapid application design were scheduled, but the clinical review organization had never been included in the current state documentation or future state visioning. Clearly, they were a key stakeholder, as a patient's file would be forwarded to them for review, and their disposition of the case would need to be routed back to the member services organization to close out the case and inform the member of the results. It is the responsibility of a process analyst or project manager to alert key project sponsors when this kind of oversight is discovered and to engage the overlooked stakeholders in the remainder of the project. This is not always easy to schedule, and there may be animosity on the part of the party that has been excluded. It is, therefore, critical to interview as many individuals as possible at the outset of a project and to ensure that all appropriate stakeholders are invited to be involved.

Conducting Interviews

The best way to fully understand the process and the stakeholders is to conduct interviews, which is a qualitative form of data collection. It is always best to start with the primary process owner—the individual with the most complete high level understanding of the flow of a process. Often a process is cross-functional, with several process owners, so it is best to begin with the process owner who has been most closely aligned with the system implementation project (i.e., the project sponsor, or the project requestor). During the interview process, ask key questions, such as:

- Who else is involved with this process?
- Is there anyone else you think I should be talking to about this process?

Process-Modeling Joint Sessions

A process can certainly be documented in pieces, as different process users are interviewed but, if it is clear whom the process involves, it is expedient to bring all of the stakeholders into a room and facilitate documentation of the process. This can be done manually, getting all of the users engaged in documenting their process using Post-it notes on flowchart paper. It can also be done with a projected process flow and one key documenter, who is able to move the process boxes around, as process steps are added and moved. It is always productive to get people energized as they move around the room, but it can be very expedient to document the process live, which eliminates time required to input the process information after the fact. However the process gets documented, the flow should include process steps that present risks or clear process improvement opportunities. The group process-modeling sessions can be used instead of or in combination with individual interviews.

COMMUNICATION PLANNING

Once it is very clear who is impacted by the process and how the process might change (improvement opportunities), it is important to begin detailed communication planning as described in Chapter 5. A good communication plan will include a stakeholder assessment, which will look at key stakeholders, the interests of those stakeholders, and the best methods for communicating with those stakeholders. Once that is understand, the plan should focus on

1. The message to be conveyed
2. The audience for each message
3. The timing of the message (i.e., when the message should be communicated or at what intervals)
4. The media, or communication vehicle
5. The person responsible for delivering the communications

While this may seem obvious and elementary, many projects I have witnessed over the years neither create nor manage a communication plan. Communication planning is a very iterative process. Communication plans need to be continuously updated throughout the life of the project.

SOLIDIFYING THE PROCESS IMPROVEMENT APPROACH

Once the current state process has been documented and analyzed for improvement opportunities, the organization should solidify its approach to process improvement. A process might give rise to a full-blown "process redesign," which would significantly change the current process or, alternatively, a more focused improvement targeted at the **low-hanging fruit**—those process steps that are the least costly and complex to rapidly improve. Once it is determined which of those two approaches will be taken, the organization should determine the methodology to use – Lean/Six Sigma, old fashioned process improvement, or some other approach. For a focused improvement, the Lean approach to conducting a one-week rapid improvement event, or Kaizen, could be useful. This is an approach similar to General Electric's "Workout™." In the Workout approach, all stakeholders and managers are brought together to work through and identify work improvements. Managers are required to approve or disapprove the desired changes (with explanation) and the approved changes are implemented within a short window of time. With a Kaizen event, the proposed changes are put into place as soon as the following week. For larger scale process improvement, old fashioned process improvement is useful.

CREATING THE FUTURE STATE

Several steps are involved in creating the future state. These include the actual visioning of the future state, as well as gap analysis between current and future states, validation of system functionality, communications and marketing of the future state.

Visioning the Solution

Designing a future state process is similar to documenting the current state. Stakeholders should meet in a room with an objective facilitator, who will encourage creativity and out-of-the-box thinking. It is always good to have people put their ideal process on Post-it notes on a flowchart. It is also fun to put people into teams and have each team present its ideal process to the other teams. The objective of the team exercise should be to increase the efficiency of the process, or create a process that enables better data capture, or improved patient care. After a team exercise, the group can jointly bring in the best ideas from all of the teams to create a common best practice process. If the current process clearly documented risks and improvement opportunities, these serve as a springboard for design of the future process.

The facilitator might target (1) mitigating existing risk followed by (2) improvement opportunities as the starting point for the process redesign. It is useful to have a software subject matter expert in the room who understands the capabilities of the system to be implemented and who can lend clarity to questions about what the application can do to enable the future state process. For example, if the current process involves a step during which the user prints a document and gets up from his or her chair to get an interoffice envelope in which to mail the document, the team might decide that an auto-send or alert feature will simplify the process. It is useful to know whether the system is going to auto-send the document or an alert, or whether another solution is required. The goal of future state design is always a more efficient and productive process. Figure 6-4 provides an example of the future process for a managed care appeals and grievances process.

There are several process improvements identified in the future state workflow in this figure. These are all improvements realized by automating the process, or including new system functionality. For example, in the current state workflow, the member

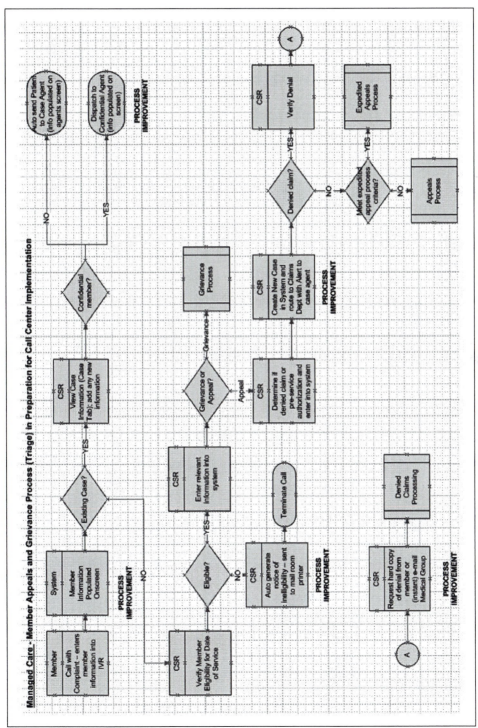

Figure 6-4: Future State of Managed Care Appeals Process

calls into the member services call center, and the customer service representative (CSR) obtains member information and enters it into the system in order to pull up that member's record. In the new call center system, the member will have entered his or her medical record number (MRN) upon dialing in to the member services center (verbally or by entering numbers on the phone touch pad). That member's information will auto-populate the CSR's computer screen, saving look-up time, and avoiding the risk of pulling up information on the wrong member, if there are two members with the same name. In another process step, instead of creating a new hard copy file, the file is created in the system and auto-routed to the next agent for processing.

The case will then arrive in the case agent's queue, and the case agent receives an alert that the case is there for processing. This saves processing time for the agent, as well as paper. It also saves the wait time previously incurred while the case was being routed interoffice. Figure 6-4 is an example of a system-driven process improvement and not a radical process improvement or redesign. In this example, the core process was not changed significantly, but improvements would be achieved through automation. There are processes, however, that will lend themselves to a more radical process redesign. The analysis phase of the project will hopefully uncover whether a process needs to be redesigned. Clues that a process needs to change considerably include patient, physician, or employee dissatisfaction, redundancy, considerable number of errors or long wait times between process steps.

Secure Buy-In

Once a new process has been identified and documented, that process needs to be "shopped" and marketed to key stakeholders and process users for validation and input. The people most impacted by the process need to understand and support the change, understanding how it will impact their workflow. There will always be trepidation, and that is where a gap analysis comes in. The gap analysis, discussed next, will indicate how to address that trepidation. The communication plan will also be instrumental in identifying the message and media to be employed in communicating the message of change.

Identify Metrics and Information Capture Points

Once the future state has been designed and buy-in secured, a few more steps must be completed before the project team can begin the process of identifying detailed system requirements. The desired metrics have to be aligned with the process steps. For example, in the process identified here, you would capture the time required to process a member's appeal, especially as the Department of Managed Healthcare specifies a required turnaround time. To capture that information, you would look at the date of the member's first contact with the health plan and the date the case is closed. It is likely you would also measure the disposition of the case, which is likely one data field. In other words, you may want to understand how often appeals are denied or overturned. If appeals are frequently overturned, it might indicate that the initial claims adjudication process is flawed. Interestingly, data captured in one process may provide insights into another related process and point to additional improvement opportunities. In this process example, it might also be useful to tie the case disposition to disease codes, physicians, clinical reviewers or any number of other data points. This should all be determined as part of the future state design.

If metrics are not considered up front, it could take significant time post-implementation to determine how to capture the required data.

Gap Analysis and System Requirements Definition

A gap analysis looks at the current state process step and the future state process step and identifies the people, process and technology gaps to get from current to future. A people gap looks at how peoples' skills need to change, how people need to be trained or how people might react to the change. A process change identifies how the process and its related activities/steps differ. A technology change indicates what the new technology will need to do to support the process, or how the new technology differs from the current technology. Figure 6-5 shows a sample gap analysis template for the process identified in the earlier figures.

System Requirements Definition

The technology gaps identified during the gap analysis will feed right into system requirements, whereas the people and process gaps will feed into the design of training materials and necessary communications required to secure buy-in. Every organization seems to have a different template, or methodology for gathering system requirements. I would propose that the best one to use is whichever approach best allows the system developers to build the application to specifications. In the past, when I have worked interactively with developers, I have found it useful to provide a template that ties requirements to each process step. That way, if the development team is unable to fulfill a requirement, it is very easy to go back to the process step impacted, and work with the process team to identify a modified process, or to propose a modification to the development team. I mention system requirements in this chapter on process improvement to ensure that it is clear that the steps of process improvement precede the system requirements definition process. It is certainly possible to develop system requirements without any focus on process, and I would conjecture that it often occurs that way. However, that is what results in a system design that does not support or transform the process that is impacted.

If a project team assesses current state, designs future state and identifies the gaps between the two, the system requirements it identifies will support the future process and address the gaps between the future and current process. Too often, a process team throws the requirements "over the wall" to the developer and the system is designed without further input from the process team. I strongly recommend that the system design be an iterative and interactive process between the developers and process team or process owners. A **rapid application design** approach (or **prototyping** as it is sometimes called), in which the users and developers are in the room together, is ideal, if your process resources' time can be made available and if the technology supports that approach. The advantage to keeping the process team engaged throughout system development is that, often, it is discovered that the system cannot do everything it was assumed that it could do. At that point, it might be necessary to modify the process

Process: Managed Care Member Appeals and Grievances

Current State Activity/Practice	Future State or Best Practice	Gap		
		PEOPLE	PROCESS	TECHNOLOGY
Call with Complaint (Grievance or Appeal)	Call with Complaint – enters member information into IVR	Member required to know his/her MRN or to enter phone number or social security number into IVR (interactive voice response unit) Training Required.	Shifts identification of member from CSR to member. Saves CSR look up time.	Need working IVR and ACD (Automated Caller Device) to recognize the member by their phone number of information entered.
Search for member information	Member Information Populated Onscreen	CSR no longer has to search menus to find member information	Process eliminated.	The required technology (IVR and ACD) need to auto-populate member information onto the CSR's screen.
Determine Case Status	(No process Step)	CSR only needs to look up case status on Case Screen. Case managers need to update case statuses; Case managers need to be trained in the new process.	Policies and procedures need to be established for documentation and updating of case statuses by the case agent.	A case status field needs to be included in the system, and it needs to be visible to the CSR.
Open Case and add Notes	View Case Information (Case Tab); add any new information	CSR does not need create a hard copy case. CSR needs to write notes into the system instead of case file. Training required.	Instead of opening a new hard copy case, an electronic case is created in the system.	System needs to contain an electronic case with imaged documents in it.
Dispatch to Case Owner and end call	Auto send Patient to Case Agent (Info populated on agents screen)	CSR doesn't need to pull a file and have it routed interoffice to the agent managing the case. Training Required.	24-48 hour interoffice transport time eliminated as case is auto-dispatched.	Documents need to be scanned and viewable in the system in order for cases to be electronic and routed.

Figure 6-5: Gap Analysis Template

given the constraints of the system. It is only in very rare circumstances that the future state process, as originally conceived, will remain 100% intact.

SUMMARY

System implementation has the ability to automate an existing process or to transform the process. If no attention is paid to process improvement in the early phase of the implementation project, the system will merely automate the existing process. Sadly, many existing processes are flawed. By automating an existing process, the ability to improve that process in the future will be hampered by the new system design. Inevitably, thousands, or even millions of dollars were spent on the system implementation, and little, if any, management support for making any changes that will impact the new system will exist. Often, when a system is implemented without a focus on process, significant costs are incurred after the fact, bringing in high-paid consultants to analyze "what went wrong" and to redefine processes that will justify the expense created during the implementation.

The phrase "pay now or pay later" applies to system implementation. By focusing on process, an organization will pay now for the resources required to ensure the process is optimal and supported by the new system. By not including process improvement as part of the implementation, the organization will pay later, not only for consultants, but also for system developers and sometimes even a brand new system or a new project team. In the latter case, the organization may be paying double or even triple the initial cost of the implementation, especially if the first implementation is abandoned. Process improvement in system implementation is not complex. It is a straightforward process involving process documentation, analysis, future visioning, gap analysis and communication and change management planning. It requires that the process team and system developers work together. Ensuring that process improvement is part of an implementation supports user adoption and eliminates project overages and post-project expense attempting to fix everything that was not addressed during implementation. Process improvement is a little bit of work that eliminates a lot of future pain.

Reference

1.   Alter A. CIOs rank their top priorities for 2008. *CIO Insight.* December 20, 2007.

SECTION III

ENGINEERING METHODS FOR PERFORMANCE IMPROVEMENT

Up to this point, we have shown how processes and projects influence performance and how management engineer or performance analysts can positively influence performance through workflow restructuring, simplification and redesign. In Part III, we describe several specific engineering methods that are useful for achieving specific results.

In Chapter 7, Kevin Roche and James Broyles, PhD students in Industrial Engineering at Arizona State University, will describe how queuing theory can be used to understand patient wait time behavior, and influence these behaviors through models by varying components of the service process (e.g., increasing the number of employees, or servers). Queuing theory has become especially valuable for projects that involve reducing cycle times in key resource-constrained areas, such as the emergency department and the operating room.

In Chapter 8, Roche and Broyles discuss simulation modeling. Similar in some regards to queuing, simulation helps to play "what if" by modeling behaviors of activities and events in a process for purposes of making improvements and changes.

In Chapter 9, John Hansmann (an immediate past member of the HIMSS Board of Directors and a long-time management engineer) describes productivity management. Understanding the relationship between inputs and outputs, and holding service lines accountable for provider and staff productivity levels, is one way that modern health systems are positively influencing overall performance. Management engineers are frequently called on to perform productivity analyses, so understanding the underlying concepts and formulas is a necessary building block.

CHAPTER 7

Queuing Theory in Healthcare

Kevin T. Roche and James R. Broyles

> *"Quality has to be caused, not controlled."*
>
> — Phil Crosby, quality guru

INTRODUCTION

Healthcare is a competitive industry in which facilities must strive to make the most of their constrained capacity. Many healthcare service systems can be viewed as queues, or waiting lines. **Queuing theory** is the science of waiting in line. In a queue, entities, typically patients in healthcare, arrive to receive some type of service or treatment. Examples of entities and systems in healthcare include patients in an emergency department, patients in an outpatient clinic, prescription requests in a hospital pharmacy, and insurance claims in an insurance company. Any time an entity (patient, request, claim) arrives, waits to be serviced, is serviced and leaves the system, the system can be viewed as a queue. This chapter provides tools that help organizations model these queuing systems to answer questions about levels of service capacity, waiting times and busyness.

   Queuing theory and simulation (simulation will be discussed in the next chapter) are useful in helping an organization properly align its service capacity with the demands of its customers. They assist an organization in modeling the effects of system changes, such as capacity and service processes, to examine its performance before implementing changes. Queuing theory uses formula-based models that can be developed at a low cost. **Simulation** is a computer-based modeling technique used as an abstract representation of a real system with an ability to be used to model very complex systems. Both simulation and queuing theory provide a structured method for solving difficult capacity allocation problems. Applying queuing theory and simulation methods provide an improved insight into the system being analyzed, along with an understanding of the following:

- The tradeoff between capacity costs and customer service
- The effect of process variability on system performance
- The correct resource utilization level for its system

When using queuing or simulation modeling, it is recommended that you work with someone who is familiar with queuing or simulation.

TYPES OF QUEUING SYSTEMS

Many types of queuing systems exist, including a single queue, multiple queue, queues in series and networks. Before the queue can be modeled or analyzed, its characteristics must be understood. Each characteristic will be discussed next.

Single Queue

One type of queuing system is a single queue system, such as that shown in Figure 7-1. A single queue system has entities that arrive, wait in a single area, get serviced by one of multiple (c) servers, and leave the system.

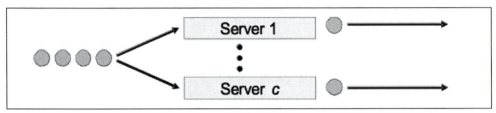

Figure 7-1: Single Queue with Multiple Servers

Single-queue, multiple-server systems are commonly used for cashier services in electronics stores, which have a line in which all customers wait before being checked out by one of the multiple cashiers.

Multiple Queues

Another type of system is a multiple queue system as shown in Figure 7-2. In this system, the entity selects a queue to enter to await service. The entity receives a service and then leaves the system.

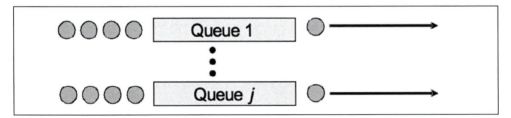

Figure 7-2: Multiple Queue System with Multiple Waiting Lines

A real-life example of multiple queues is observable at the grocery store, with a line (or queue) at each cashier. This setup is actually less efficient than the single-line, multiple-server queuing system but can easily be implemented in waiting space constrained areas that cannot support a long, single line.

Queues in Series

Some systems can be considered as queues in series. In this system, all entities receive service from sequential server queues in the same order. In Figure 7-3, the entity awaits server 1 in Queue 1 before proceeding to await server 2 in Queue 2, and so on. Queues in series frequently exist for situations in which each entity in the system uses resources in the same manner. For example, all trucks on an automotive assembly line are routed sequentially to the same stations for service.

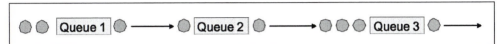

Figure 7-3: A Multiple Queues in Series System

Queuing Network

Sometimes multiple queues are not visited sequentially (or by all entities), as shown in Figure 7-4. In queuing networks, entities are routed probabilistically from one queue to the next. In Figure 7-4, once entities are finished receiving service from Queue 1, some entities go directly to Queue 2, with some probability and some go directly to Queue 3, with another probability.

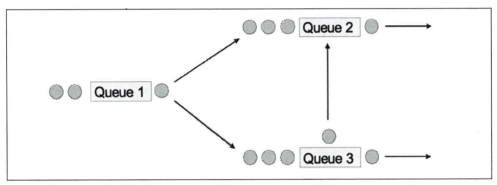

Figure 7-4: A Network of Queues

Queuing networks come in many different configurations. Some feed backward, resulting in re-entrant flow. An example of re-entrant flow could be seen in Figure 7-4, if Queue 3 had sent some entities back to Queue 1 after service. An emergency department in a hospital might be viewed as a queuing network, as different entities (patients) require different resources (treatments).

THE ARRIVAL AND SERVICE PROCESSES

Two very important characteristics of a queuing system are the arrival and service processes. To discuss these processes, let us first define an arrival event, a start-of-service event, and an end-of-service event. An **arrival event** occurs when an entity arrives to the system. A **start-of-service event** occurs when the entity subsequently begins service. Finally, the **end-of-service event** arises when the entity finishes service, and the server is freed. By recording the time of each of these events, average time between

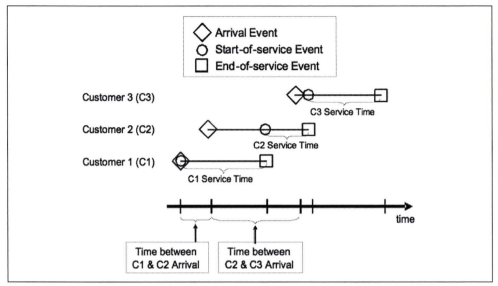

Figure 7-5: Depiction of Event Times, Time between Arrivals, and Service Times

arrivals and average service time per server can be calculated. Both of these calculations are important inputs to any queuing theory or computer simulation model. To better identify how these calculations are derived, consider the following example:

Suppose an outpatient clinic has a single treatment room and, therefore, can treat only one patient at a time. This queuing system is a single queue system (recall Figure 7-1) with one server (c = 1).

Figure 7-5 shows the arrival and service events for three patients.

Recording and collecting the times of these three events for each entity facilitates the calculation of the average time between arrivals and average service time. As a side note, the time between the arrival event and the start-of-service event is the time spent waiting.

Using the average time between arrivals (A) and the average service time per entity (B), the calculation of the arrival rate λ (lambda) and the service rate μ (mu) are shown in the following calculation:

$$\lambda = \left(A\right)^{-1} = \frac{1}{A} \qquad\qquad \mu = \left(B\right)^{-1} = \frac{1}{B}$$

The units of the arrival rate λ and the service rate μ are patients per time unit. For example, if $A = 10$ minutes and $B = 9$ minutes, $\lambda = 0.1$ patients per minute and $\mu = 0.11$ patients per minute. It is essential to use consistent time units for both A and B (hours, minutes, etc.) in any queuing analysis.

WHY DO QUEUES FORM?

Queues, or waiting lines, form due to randomness in the arrival and service processes. Typically, the time between arrivals and the service times are random variables in that they are not the same duration for every customer. This randomness is called **variability.** To illustrate, let us look at a counterexample.

Suppose patients arrive to an outpatient clinic that has only one physician. Also, suppose that the time between patient arrivals is always *exactly* 10 minutes and the treatment time per patient is *exactly* 9 minutes. The physician will be occupied 9 of every 10 minutes (physician utilization = 9/10 = 90%) and no queue will form. Now suppose that the time between patient arrivals varies randomly between 5 and 15 minutes with an average of 10 minutes and the service time varies randomly between 4 and 14 minutes with an average of 9 minutes. This physician will be occupied on average 9 of every 10 minutes (physician utilization = 90%) but, this time, a queue will eventually form because some patients will arrive before the previous service is completed. In general, more variability in a system's arrival and service processes increases waiting.

The Role of Variability on Throughput

As mentioned previously, variability in the arrival and service processes can lead to delays and waiting. One measure of variability is the **coefficient of variation (cv).** The cv of any distribution is equal to the standard deviation divided by the mean:

$$Coefficient\ of\ Variation\ (cv)\ = \frac{Standard\ deviation}{Mean}$$

When the cv approaches or exceeds 1.0, variability is quite large and can significantly affect the system.

Figure 7-6 shows how variability affects patient waiting times. As the expected wait time climbs from under 10 minutes to over 45 minutes, the only change occurring is an increase in service time variability. The system is still seeing the same raw number of patients per time unit, and these patients still have the same *average* service time. Six Sigma methodologies, discussed earlier in Chapter 4, focus on standardization and variability reduction to benefit system operations.

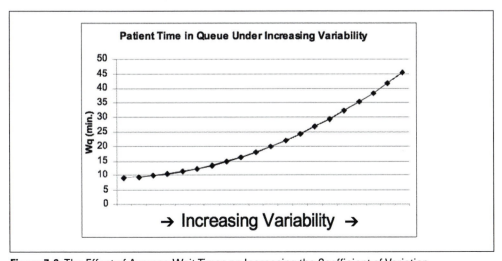

Figure 7-6: The Effect of Average Wait Times on Increasing the Coefficient of Variation

WHEN TO APPLY QUEUING THEORY OR SIMULATION

In general, the decision whether to use queuing theory or simulation is left to the modeler. Although simulation will be more thoroughly discussed in the next chapter, let's discuss the primary differences here. The modeler must be aware of the assumptions and consequences of choosing either. Queuing theory and simulation both have advantages and disadvantages. The modeler must attempt to select the one that provides the modeling power needed, knowing fully the modeling resource requirements and the assumptions of the technique selected. Let's first look at the modeling assumptions, then the modeling resources required and finally compare the advantages and disadvantages of both queuing theory and simulation.

There are several fundamental modeling assumptions made when applying queuing theory that simulation does not require. Queuing theory assumes the arrival rate λ, service rate μ, and service capacity c are all **stationary**, meaning that, although variation may be present, the mean of a process does not change with time. This assumption might not be correct in the real system. In computer simulation, λ, μ, and c are not required to be stationary and can change according to the coder's request. With that said, sometimes systems that do not have constant rates or service capacity can be approximated using queuing theory.

For example, Banner Health created a queuing system of its emergency departments, which experience non-stationary arrival rates (Figure 7-7).[1] In addition, service capacity was not stationary because more staff would be present during the afternoon and evening than in the morning. However, they realized that their staffing capacity and arrival rate were fairly stationary from 9:00 a.m. to 9:00 p.m. (peak period) every day. Since the major concern of the modeling effort was to appropriately capacitate the ED during the peak period, a queuing model was built that analyzed only the peak period of the day. If that organization wanted to model every hour of the day with a customized staffing pattern, computer simulation would be necessary.

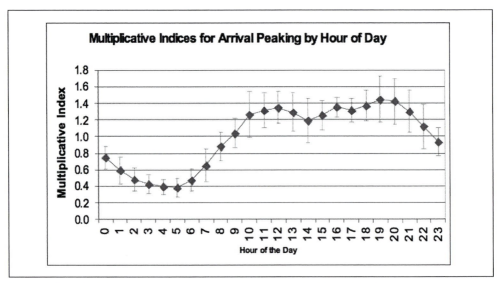

Figure 7-7: Arrival Rate to a Hospital Emergency Department by Hour of the Day

A number of other queuing-based analytical approximations can help to overcome the problems of non-stationarity. For example, Stolletz[2] introduced the Stationary Backlog Carryover (SBC) approach, which provides performance measures for non-stationary systems, even when utilization is more than 100% for some time. The SBC approach is compared with some of the other approximations and is shown to meet or exceed their performance when compared with simulation.

The modeling resources required between queuing theory and simulation are vastly different. Queuing theory requires the use of mathematical calculations and, as a result, can be implemented in any spreadsheet software that allows the use of formulas. In fact, there are several free spreadsheet-based queuing software packages that will calculate the formulas presented in the rest of this chapter. On the other hand, simulation software usually requires a license for the commercial simulation package. In addition, an organization needs to have someone who knows how to use and interpret the inputs and outputs of that simulation package. Because a simulation model is highly customizable, much data must be collected from the real system to input into the simulation.

With these assumptions and the modeling resource requirements in mind, there are clear benefits and drawbacks to both queuing theory and simulation. Some of these are highlighted in Table 7-1.

Table 7-1: Benefits and Drawbacks of Queuing and Simulation

	Benefits	Drawbacks
Queuing	Analytical results; Requires no output analysis; Formulas can be used in a spreadsheet; Can be generic; No cost!	Not as flexible as simulation; Does not always provide distributions on W_q, W, L_q, L
Simulation	Very flexible; Situational specific; Can model complex systems; Estimates distributions on W_q, W, L_q, L for all systems	Requires experimental design and analysis; Requires a simulation package; Expensive in both capital and time; Need to decide run lengths, replications, and statistical significance; Not generic

Although not an analytical technique, discrete-event simulation (DES) modeling can be very useful in modeling complex systems with non-stationary arrival and service processes, complex entity flow and time-dependant system capacity. Although DES provides some advantages over queuing, there are also some disadvantages to consider.

Instead of predicting system performance analytically through formulas, DES relies on averages of system performance over a simulated time horizon. Simulation requires the purchase (and licensing) of a simulation software package. Additionally, an organization must have someone who is familiar with the package and can build complex models. The following chapter will discuss this in more detail. While queuing theory cannot model very complicated systems and makes assumptions about process stationarity, it is inexpensive and fairly easy to use.

System Performance Measures

The main outputs of any model using either queuing theory or computer simulation are the system performance measures. Some of the most important long-term system performance measures are:

- *Utilization* (ρ): the average fraction of time the queuing system's servers are busy.
- *Probability of an Empty System* (p_0): the fraction of time the system is empty.
- *Probability of n Patients in the System* (p_n): the fraction of time there are exactly *n* entities in the system.
- *Average Number of Entities in the System* (L): the average number of entities in service and in the queue (units = number of patients).
- *Average Number of Entities in the Queue* (L_q): the average number of entities waiting in the queue (units = number of patients).
- *Average Time in System* (W): the average time an entity spends in the system. Time in the system includes time waiting in the queue and time spent in service (units = time).
- *Average Time in Queue* (W_q): the average time an entity spends waiting for service (units = time).

Queuing theory uses formulas that calculate these performance measures. Computer simulation determines these performance measures by collecting observations.

There are no definitive rules for picking target performance measures when designing a system; instead, target system performance is unique to each modeling situation. In reality, choosing the right service capacity is a function of both performance and cost. When modeling, it is important to understand the relationships between these performance measures.

When measuring system utilization, for example, it is important to note the non-linear relationship between utilization and both time in system and waiting time. When applied to a modeling exercise, an analyst must understand that although high utilizations are desirable from a financial perspective, they can hurt system performance because high utilizations result in extremely long waiting times. Figure 7-8 illustrates that system utilization has a much larger effect on waiting time at higher utilization levels.

Increasing utilization from 65% to 70% has a far smaller impact on wait times (Wq) than increasing utilization from 90% to 95%.

Because the 'right' system performance is a trade-off between finances and capacity, it is important to quantify the potential costs in the system. Consider the example of an emergency department (ED) manager. She wishes to keep small wait times for arriving patients to be initially screened by a triage nurse. Modeling the screening process as a queuing system with nurses as servers, the manager must trade off the expense of staffed nursing hours with the expense of patient waiting to keep overall system costs low. Figure 7-9 illustrates the cost trade-off.

Although it is desirable from a service standpoint to see patients quickly, keeping system utilization low enough to maintain good wait times means a higher cost of service.

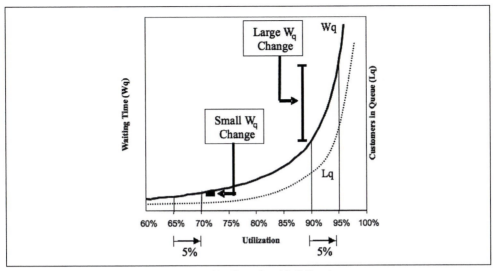

Figure 7-8: Expected Wait Times Increase Nonlinearly with Utilization

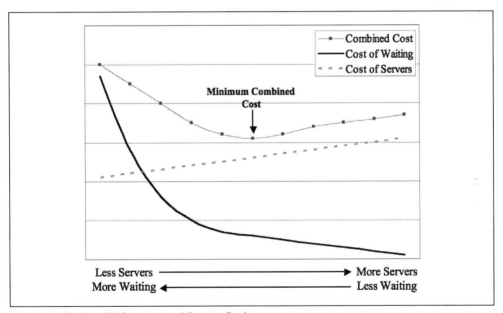

Figure 7-9: Trading Off Capacity and System Performance

THE MODELING PROCESS

Whether queuing theory or simulation is selected to model a system, the modeling process in both is similar. The steps of modeling a queuing system follow.

Step 1: Define the Problem and Gather Data

Take a look at the whole queuing system. Draw a system diagram similar to the ones seen in Figures 7-1 through 7-4. Some example systems in healthcare include hospital bed units, surgery suites, outpatient clinics, and call centers. A common modeling goal of these systems would be to define the capacity necessary to operate 'efficiently.' Efficiency can be measured through server utilization, expected entity wait times, expected entity loss, etc. depending on the characteristics of the problem and the system. Once the problem has been defined, relevant data must be gathered to support analysis of the system. For example, if the system in question is an outpatient clinic, the important data would include patient arrival and service times, as well as current system capacity and performance.

Step 2: Formulate a Model

Once data have been collected and analyzed, a model of the system can be developed. As discussed earlier, the type of queuing or simulation model to be implemented depends on the characteristics of the situation under analysis. Model classification and selection will be discussed in depth in this chapter.

Step 3: Validate Model Inputs and Outputs

Essential to any modeling effort is **validation,** which is the act of ensuring that the model accurately reflects the real system. Input data must be validated against the actual performance of the system being modeled. This is accomplished in a number of ways, including a comparison of input parameters to actual data and a discussion of input data with staff who are intimately familiar with the real system. Once the data have been validated and input into the model, the output of the model must be validated. To ensure that the model matches reality, the output performance measures should be compared with those from the system under analysis. Are the measures within acceptable ranges, or are there significant differences? If differences exist and are significant, the model should be re-examined and step 2 should be repeated until the source of error is identified and the gap in performance measures is closed.

Step 4: Implement Model and Evaluate Scenarios

Once the model has been proven valid, and it accurately mimics the real-life system, it is now safer to evaluate hypothetical scenarios with the model. For example, if patient arrival volume is expected to increase, increase the volume in the model to view the effect on system performance measures of interest. At this stage, the analyst can experiment with system capacity or process changes to evaluate the impact of these hypothetical changes.

APPLICATION OF QUEUING THEORY

The mathematics behind queuing were developed in the early 1900s by A.K. Erlang, a mathematician interested in quantifying performance measures of a telephone traffic system.[3] Since his early research, the use of queuing has grown and researchers have discovered new formulations that can solve many diverse and difficult problems.

The remainder of this section provides the reader with the basic tools needed to apply queuing theory and analyze queuing systems. First, probability distributions are discussed to provide the reader with a basis for modeling. Next, the standard queuing notation is defined, and finally, formulations and examples are presented for some basic queue types.

Probability Distributions and Kendall's Notation

In 1953, David Kendall created a standard notation for the purpose of labeling types of queues. To understand the notation, we must first discuss probability distributions with respect to the arrival and service process. The two most important probability distributions in queuing theory are the exponential and Poisson distributions. Let the random variables I and S represent the time between arrival events (inter-arrival time) and service time, respectively. As discussed earlier, the average of I is $1/\lambda$, and the average of S is $1/\mu$. If I and S were exponentially distributed, they would have a probability density function that looks like Figure 7-10.

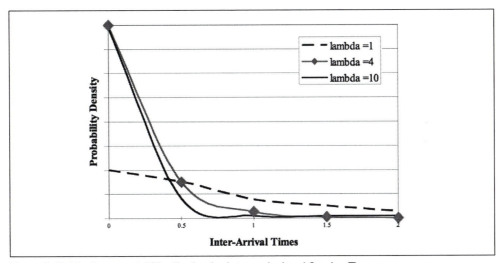

Figure 7-10: The Exponential Distribution for Inter-arrival and Service Times

One way to check if they are exponentially distributed is to create a histogram of inter-arrival and service time data. In addition, check that the I's and S's standard deviations are nearly equal to their averages; we know from probability theory the standard deviation of an exponential distribution equals the average. If the histogram looks similar to one of the graphs in Figure 7-10, and the standard deviation is very close to the mean (coefficient of variation $\cong$ 1), assuming an exponential distribution would not be a bad assumption.

If your inter-arrival time and service times are exponentially distributed with means $1/\lambda$ and $1/\mu$, respectively, we know from probability theory that the arrival and service rates are Poisson distributed with means λ and μ, respectively. The Poisson distribution has units of counts per time unit and is shown in Figure 7-11 for different means.

Once the distribution of arrival and service processes is known, Kendall's notation (defined next) can be used to describe different queue types.

Kendall's notation is a simple notation scheme that displays information about the arrival and service distribution types, the number of servers (c), and the system capacity (K). Some queuing systems have a maximum number of entities that can be in the system at any time; any additional arrivals when the system is full are lost. The maximum number of entities in the system (K) is the number of servers (c) plus the maximum number of spaces in the queue. If *K* is omitted in Kendall's notation, it is assumed there is infinite system capacity. Kendall's notation is described in Figure 7-12.

For example, an M/M/1 queue has exponential inter-arrival and service distributions with one server and an infinite capacity. An M/M/4/10 queue has exponential inter-arrival and service distributions with c=4 servers and a system capacity of K=10. An M/G/2 queue has an exponential inter-arrival time distribution, a general service distribution, c=2 servers, and an infinite system capacity; we will discuss a general distribution in more detail later.

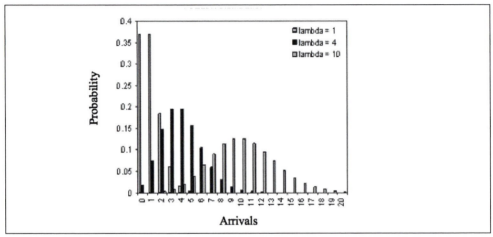

Figure 7-11: The Poisson Distribution for Arrival and Service Rates

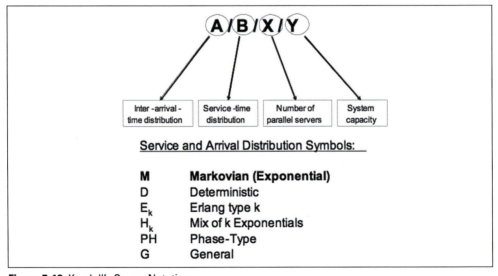

Figure 7-12: Kendall's Queue Notation

GENERAL RESULTS FOR ALL QUEUES WITH INFINITE CAPACITY

Kendall's notation allows us to distinguish between different types of queues. With that said, there exist general performance measures that apply to all queue types with infinite system capacity ($K=\infty$). These performance measures are displayed in Table 7-2.

Table 7-2 is divided into three types: data, model input, and performance calculation. Data are the information obtained from collecting data from the real-life system. Model inputs are the number of servers and the system capacity that the modeler wants to evaluate. Performance calculations are the outputs from the queuing model. The elements in this table are valid for any type of infinite capacity queue except for p_0 and p_n. p_0 and p_n are dependent on the queuing system being modeled and will be described in the following sections. Later, you will also see that p_n will be used to calculate L and L_q.

Table 7-2: General Inputs and Performance Measure for Queues

Type	Name	Symbol	Calculation	Units
Data	Average Time Between Arrivals	A		time
	Average Service Time	S		time
Model Input	Number of Servers	c		servers
	System Capacity	K		customers
Performance Calculation	Arrival Rate	λ (lambda)	$= 1/A$	customers/time
	Service Rate	μ (mu)	$= 1/S$	customers/time
	Average Number of Busy Servers	r	$= \lambda/\mu$	servers
	Server Utilization	ρ (rho)	$= r/c = \lambda/(c\,\mu)$	
	Probability of Empty System	p_0	queue type dependant	
	Probability of n Customers in the System	p_n	queue type dependant	
	Average Number of Customers in the System	L	$= \lambda\,W = L_q + r$	customers
	Average Number of Customers in the Queue	L_q	$= \lambda\,W_q = L - r$	customers
	Average Total Time in the System per Customer	W	$= W_q + 1/\mu = L/\lambda$	time
	Average Waiting Time in the System per Customer	W_q	$= W - 1/\mu = L_q/\lambda$	time

QUEUE TYPES AND PERFORMANCE MEASURES

The next sections contain a list of queue types and performance measures. When performing queuing analysis, it is important that all time units are the same (for example all in hours). Mixing time units for the arrival and service processes can lead to misleading performance outputs.

The final section of this chapter discusses available software that will automatically compute all equations in the following models. The formulations are presented in this chapter to provide the reader with the background for queuing analysis and guidelines for simple calculations.

M/M/1 Queue

An M/M/1 queue system has exponential inter-arrival and service times with a single server and infinite system capacity. Figure 7-1 shown earlier depicts the M/M/1 queue. Utilization (ρ) must be less than 1 in order to calculate any performance measure. M/M/1 performance measures can be calculated as follows:

$$p_0 = 1 - \rho \qquad\qquad p_n = (1 - \rho)\rho^n$$

$$L = \frac{\lambda}{\mu - \lambda} \qquad L_q = \frac{\lambda^2}{\mu(\mu - \lambda)} \qquad W = \frac{1}{\mu - \lambda} \qquad W_q = \frac{\rho}{\mu - \lambda}$$

Example: Customers arrive to a single physician clinic that can treat only one patient at a time (c=1). Time between patient arrivals is exponentially distributed (M) with average 0.5 hours (A = 0.5 hours) and service times are exponentially distributed (M) with average 24 minutes (S = 24 minutes = 0.4 hours). What is the long-run average number of patients waiting (L_q), and how long does a patient wait on average (W_q)?

Answer: This single physician clinic is an M/M/1 queuing system with arrival rate $\lambda = 1/A = 1/0.5 = 2$ patients per hour and service rate $\mu = 1/S = 1/0.4 = 2.5$ patients per hour. Therefore, server utilization $\rho = \lambda/(c \times \mu) = 2/(1 \times 2.5) = 0.8$, the average number of patients waiting $Lq = \lambda^2/(\mu(\mu - \lambda)) = 2^2/(2.5 \times (2.5-2)) = 3.2$ patients, and the average waiting time $W_q = \rho/(\mu - \lambda) = 0.8/(2.5-2) = 1.6$ hours.

M/M/c Queue

An M/M/c queue system is the multi-server version of and M/M/1. Figure 7-1 shown earlier depicts the M/M/c queue. Again, utilization (ρ) must be less than 1. Performance measures for the M/M/c queue are as follows:

$$p_0 = \left(\sum_{n=0}^{c-1} \frac{r^n}{n!} + \frac{r^c}{c!(1-\rho)} \right)^{-1} \qquad p_n = \begin{cases} \dfrac{\rho^n}{n!} p_0 & for\ 1 \le n < c \\[2ex] \dfrac{\rho^n}{c^{n-c}c!} p_0 & for\ n \ge c \end{cases}$$

$$L = \lambda W \qquad\qquad L_q = \left(\frac{r^c \rho}{c!(1-\rho)^2} \right) p_0$$

$$W = W_q + \frac{1}{\mu} \qquad W_q = \frac{L_q}{\lambda}$$

where x factorial (or x!) = x*(x-1)*(x-2)*...*2*1 (eg. 4! = 4*3*2*1 = 24) and 0! =1, the mathematical inverse of x (or x^{-1}) = 1/x, and the summation of 2^x from 0 to 2 (or $\sum_{x=0}^{2} 2^x$) = $2^0 + 2^1 + 2^2 = 1+2+4 = 7$.

Example: A hospital has two fully staffed and fully functional surgery rooms dedicated strictly to emergency surgery that can operate with one patient in each room (c=2). The time between arrivals is exponentially distributed (M) with an average of 120 minutes (A = 120 min = 2 hours) and the surgery times are exponentially distributed (M) with an average of 3 hours (S = 3 hours). What is the probability that there are no patients in surgery (p_0)? What is the average number of emergency surgery patients waiting for surgery (L_q)? What is the average time an emergency patient waits for surgery (W_q)?

Answer: This surgery ward is an M/M/2 queuing system with arrival rate $\lambda = 1/A = 1/2 = 0.5$ patients per hour and service rate $\mu = 1/S = 1/3 \approx 0.33$ patients per hour. Therefore, the average number of busy surgery rooms $r = \lambda/\mu = 0.5/0.33 \approx 1.52$ surgery rooms and the average server utilization $\rho = r/c = 1.52/2 = 0.76$. The probability that there are no patients in surgery (p_0) and the average number of emergency surgery patients waiting for surgery L_q are calculated as follows:

$$p_0 = \left(\sum_{n=0}^{c-1} \frac{r^n}{n!} + \frac{r^c}{c!(1-\rho)} \right)^{-1} = \left(\sum_{n=0}^{2-1} \frac{1.52^n}{n!} + \frac{1.52^2}{2!(1-0.76)} \right)^{-1} = \left(\sum_{n=0}^{1} \frac{1.52^n}{n!} + \frac{1.52^2}{(2*1)(1-0.76)} \right)^{-1}$$

$$= \left(\frac{1.52^0}{0!} + \frac{1.52^1}{1!} + 4.81 \right)^{-1} = \left(1 + 1.52 + 4.81\right)^{-1} = \left(7.33\right)^{-1} = \frac{1}{7.33} = 0.136$$

$$L_q = \left(\frac{r^c \rho}{c!(1-\rho)^2} \right) p_0 = \left(\frac{1.52^2 * 0.76}{2!(1-0.76)^2} \right) * 0.136 = \left(15.24\right) * 0.136 = 2.07 \text{ patients}$$

The average amount of time a patients waits is $W_q = L_q/\lambda = 2.07/0.5 = 4.14$ hours.

M/M/c/K Queue

An M/M/c/K queue system has exponential inter-arrival and service times with c servers and a system capacity of K. If a customer arrives and the system is full with K entities, the arrival is lost; this is called balking. **Balking** occurs when a customer arrives to find the system full and therefore leaves immediately. When there is a system capacity, a fraction of the arrivals are lost (p_K) because they find the system to be full. Therefore, the effective rate at which customers enter the queue (λ_{eff}) is the arrival rate multiplied by the probability that the queue is not full ($1-p_K$); in other words, $\lambda_{eff} = \lambda(1-p_K)$. Because entities are balked from the system, a utilization $\rho \geq 1$ is now possible. The performance measures are as follows:

$$p_0 = \begin{cases} \left[\left(\sum_{n=0}^{c-1} \frac{r^n}{n!} \right) + \left(\frac{r^c}{c!} \right) \left(\frac{1-\rho^{K-c+1}}{(1-\rho)} \right) \right]^{-1} & \text{for } \rho \neq 1 \\ \left[\sum_{n=0}^{c-1} \frac{r^n}{n!} + \left(\frac{r^c}{c!} \right) (K-c+1) \right]^{-1} & \text{for } \rho = 1 \end{cases} \qquad p_n = \begin{cases} \frac{r^n}{n!} p_0 & \text{for } 1 \leq n < c \\ \frac{r^n}{c^{n-c} c!} p_0 & \text{for } c \leq n \leq K \end{cases}$$

$$L_q = \frac{p_0 r^c \rho}{c!(1-\rho)^2} \left(1 - \rho^{K-c+1} - (1-\rho)(K-c+1)\rho^{K-c} \right)$$

$$L = L_q + \frac{\lambda_{eff}}{\mu} \qquad\qquad W = \frac{L}{\lambda_{eff}} \qquad\qquad W_q = \frac{L_q}{\lambda_{eff}}$$

A special case is M/M/1/K where there is only one server c=1. The calculations for p_0, p_n, and L_q change, but the L, W, and W_q remain the same as in the formula just presented:

$$p_0 = \begin{cases} \dfrac{1-\rho}{1-\rho^{K+1}} & \text{for } \rho \neq 1 \\[2ex] \dfrac{1}{K+1} & \text{for } \rho = 1 \end{cases} \qquad p_n = \begin{cases} \dfrac{(1-\rho)\rho^n}{1-\rho^{K+1}} & \text{for } \rho \neq 1 \\[2ex] \dfrac{1}{K+1} & \text{for } \rho = 1 \end{cases}$$

$$L_q = \begin{cases} \dfrac{\rho}{1-\rho} - \dfrac{\rho(K\rho^K+1)}{1-\rho^{K+1}} & \text{for } \rho \neq 1 \\[2ex] \dfrac{K(K-1)}{2(K+1)} & \text{for } \rho = 1 \end{cases}$$

Another special case is the pure overflow model M/M/c/c in which the system capacity is equal to the number of servers K=c. This model is called Erlang's loss model and is valid for 'pure overflow' queues, regardless of the service time distribution (M/G/c/c). In the **pure overflow system,** there is no room for waiting, and any arrivals that occur when there are already c entities in the system will be balked. Again, because arrivals are balked, a utilization $\rho \geq 1$ is allowable. Because there is no waiting, both the average length of queue and waiting time in the queue are zero ($L_q = W_q = 0$). The p_n distribution reduces to the following:

$$p_n = \frac{r^n/n!}{\sum\limits_{i=0}^{c} r^i/i!} \quad \text{for } 0 \leq n \leq c$$

Example: A hospital has 126 beds (c=126) in its intensive care unit (ICU). The time between patient arrivals is exponentially distributed (M) with an average of 24 minutes (A = 24 min. = 0.0167 days) and the patient length of stay (LOS) is exponentially distributed (M) with an average of 48 hours (S = 48 hours = 2 days). If an ICU patient arrives and all ICU beds are occupied, the patient is balked and is immediately transferred to another hospital (K=c=126). What is the probability that a patient will balk and be transferred to another hospital (p_{126})? What is the rate at which patients are balked to another hospital ($\lambda^* p_{126}$)?

Answer: This ICU is an M/M/126/126 pure overflow queuing system with arrival rate $\lambda = 1/A = 1/0.0167 = 59.9$ patients per day and a service rate $\mu = 1/S = 1/2 = 0.5$ patients per day. The probability that a patient is balked to another hospital p_{126} (or the probability of being full) is calculated using Erlang's loss model as follows:

$$p_{n=126} = \frac{r^n/n!}{\sum\limits_{i=0}^{c} r^i/i!} = \frac{119.8^{126}/126!}{\sum\limits_{i=0}^{126} 119.8^i/i!} = \frac{3.24*10^{50}}{\dfrac{119.8^0}{0!} + \dfrac{119.8^1}{1!} + ... + \dfrac{119.8^{125}}{125!} + \dfrac{119.8^{126}}{126!}} = \frac{3.24*10^{50}}{7.83*10^{51}} = 0.041$$

The rate at which patients are balked to another hospital is $\lambda * p_{126} = 59.9*0.041 = 2.46$ patients per day.

G/G/c Queue

A G/G/c queue system has general inter-arrival and service times with c servers and no system capacity. A **general distribution** is an unknown distribution that requires estimation of the mean and standard deviation. Remember, the coefficient of variation is the standard deviation divided by the mean as discussed earlier. The inter-arrival time coefficient of variation (cv_A) is the standard deviation of the inter-arrival time divided by the average inter-arrival time calculated from the collected data. Similarly, the service time coefficient of variation (cv_S) is the standard deviation of the service time divided by the average service time calculated from the collected data. Many software packages require the variance as an input instead of standard deviation; variance is simply the standard deviation squared. The G/G/c performance measures are as follows:

$$W_q = \left(\frac{r^c p_0}{c(1-\rho)^2 c!}\right)\left(\frac{cv_A^2 + cv_S^2}{2}\right)\left(\frac{1}{\mu}\right)$$

$$W = W_q + \frac{1}{\mu} \qquad L_q = \lambda W_q \qquad L = \lambda W$$

where p_0 is the M/M/c's p_0.

A G/G/1 queue system is a special case of the G/G/c system that has general inter-arrival and service times with one server (c=1) and no system capacity. The equations for the G/G/c just given can be used for the G/G/1 by setting c=1.

Example: A low acuity outpatient clinic has two treatment rooms (c=2). The time between arrivals is distributed with an unknown distribution (G) with an average of 66.7 minutes (A = 66.7 min. = 1.11 hours) and a standard deviation near 66.7 minutes (1.11 hours). The treatment time is distributed according to an unknown distribution (G) with an average of 2 hours (S = 2 hours) and a standard deviation of 1.2 hours. What is the average waiting time per customer (W_q)?

Answer: This outpatient clinic is a G/G/2 queuing system with arrival rate $\lambda = 1/A = 1/1.11 = 0.9$ patients per hour, $cv_A = 1.11/A = 1.11/1.11 = 1$, service rate $\mu = 1/S = 1/2 = 0.5$ patients per hour, and $cv_S = 1.2/S = 1.2/2 = 0.6$. Therefore, the average number of busy rooms is $r = \lambda/\mu = 0.9/0.5 = 1.8$ rooms, and the average room utilization is $\rho = \lambda/(c*\mu) = 0.9/(2*0.5) = 0.9$. To find W_q, we first need to find p_0 using the M/M/c p_0:

$$p_0 = \left(\sum_{n=0}^{c-1}\frac{r^n}{n!} + \frac{r^c}{c!(1-\rho)}\right)^{-1} = \left(\sum_{n=0}^{2-1}\frac{1.8^n}{n!} + \frac{1.8^2}{2!(1-0.9)}\right)^{-1} = \left(\sum_{n=0}^{1}\frac{1.8^n}{n!} + 16.2\right)^{-1}$$

$$= \left(\frac{1.8^0}{0!} + \frac{1.8^1}{1!} + 16.2\right)^{-1} = (1 + 1.8 + 16.2)^{-1} = (19)^{-1} = \frac{1}{19} = 0.053$$

Therefore, the average amount of time a patient must wait W_q is as follows:

$$W_q = \left(\frac{r^c p_0}{c(1-\rho)^2 c!}\right)\left(\frac{cv_A^2 + cv_S^2}{2}\right)\left(\frac{1}{\mu}\right) = \left(\frac{1.8^2 * 0.053}{2 * (1-0.9)^2 * 2!}\right)\left(\frac{1^2 + 0.6^2}{2}\right)\left(\frac{1}{0.5}\right)$$

$$= (4.293)(0.68)(2) = 5.84 \text{ hours}$$

SERIES AND NETWORKS OF M/M/c QUEUES

A series of M/M/c queues occurs when all entities sequentially visit multiple M/M/c queues. Figure 7-3 shown earlier depicts this type of queuing system. If every queue in the series has no waiting room constraint between the queues, each queue can be analyzed independently, as appropriate with the arrival rate to each queue equal to the arrival rate at the very first queue.

A network of M/M/c queues occurs when entities are routed probabilistically between multiple M/M/c queues. Figure 7-4 depicts this type of queuing system. If every queue in the network has infinite waiting space constraint between the queues, each queue can be analyzed independently. The arrival rate to each queue (λ_i) is equal to that queue's external arrival rate (γ_i), plus the summation of every other queue's arrival rate, multiplied by their transfer probability to queue i ($\Sigma(\lambda_j{}^*r_{ji})$), or

$$\lambda_i = \gamma_i + \sum_{j=1}^{n} \lambda_j * r_{ji}$$

Sometimes the assumption of infinite waiting space between queues is not valid. When this exists, entities occasionally may not enter the next queue because the next queue is full and, as a result, they are blocked in their current queue until the next queue has available system capacity. A real-life example of this occurs when admitted ED patients cannot be transferred to an inpatient hospital bed because the inpatient department lacks the capacity to admit more patients. Therefore, patients are blocked in the emergency department. If blocking exists, the queuing analysis presented in this chapter is invalid. The queuing theory analysis of blocking systems is beyond the scope of this chapter, but additional information on blocking can be found at Perros[4] and Koizumi et al.[5]

QUEUING THEORY SOFTWARE

A main benefit of queuing is the ability to be easily implemented. As a result, there are several software packages available for a low cost. Additionally, freeware, such as QTS Plus (1994) (highly recommended) and QTP (2003), is available that works on the Microsoft Excel platform and allows analysis of many queuing systems. Also, because of the analytical nature of queuing, formulae can be easily and quickly coded and implemented by a user in any spreadsheet software.

SUMMARY

The information presented in this chapter is meant to provide the reader with a high-level overview of the capabilities of queuing analysis and some useful formulae. Queuing can be used to significantly improve performance of hospitals and health systems. There is much more to learn on this subject, as alluded to throughout the section. A good text for further information on queuing theory is Gross and Harris,[6] which covers everything from standard queuing formulations to more theoretical material. In addition, Ozcan[7] takes a more applied approach to queuing and highlights applications in healthcare.

References

1. Cochran JK, Roche KR. A multi-class queuing network methodology for improving hospital emergency department performance. *Computers and Operations Research.* 2008; 2:1-16.
2. Stolletz R. Non-stationary delay analysis of runaway systems. *OR Spectrum.* 2008; 30:191-213.
3. E Brockmeyer, Halstrom HL, Jensen A. *The life and works of AK Erlang.* Copenhagen: The Copenhagen Telephone Company; 1948.
4. Perros HG. *Queuing Networks with Blocking.* Oxford University Press Inc.; 1994.
5. Koizumi N, Kuno E, Smith TE. Modeling patient flows using a queuing network with blocking. *Healthcare Management Science.* 2005; 8:49-60.
6. Gross D, Harris CM. *Fundamentals of Queuing Theory.* New York: John Wiley and Sons; 1998.
7. Ozcan YA. *Quantitative Methods in Healthcare Management: Techniques and Applications.* San Francisco: Jossey-Bass; 2005.

CHAPTER 8

Simulation Modeling in Healthcare

Kevin T. Roche and James R. Broyles

> *"Quality is not an act, it is a habit."*
>
> — Aristotle

INTRODUCTION

Simulation is another option for system modeling and analysis. Simulation is used to evaluate the changes to a model of a system over time. Because many real-life systems are too complex for the use of analytical solutions, such as queuing, simulation is used to develop good estimates for how the model will behave over time.

Unlike queuing, simulation can be employed in situations with non-stationary behaviors. This means that when there are different arrival or service patterns, or a varying service capacity, simulation can be used to model the system. As a result, simulation has been frequently used in healthcare to model systems, such as emergency departments,[1] individual bed units,[2] and whole hospitals.[3]

The topic of simulation is very broad and consequently, this chapter will focus on the basics of how simulation works, the inputs and outputs from a simulation model, verification and validation of models, a few notable simulation packages and direction for further information on the simulation modeling process.

DISCRETE-EVENT SIMULATION

The most commonly employed method of simulation to healthcare problems is discrete-event simulation (DES). In DES, changes to a system occur only at a countable number of moments in time. An example of a change in a system would be the arrival of a patient to a queue or the completion of service on a patient. This is in contrast with continuous-time simulations in which the system changes continuously over time.

Most computerized discrete-event simulators use a "next-event time advance" approach in which the times of future events are recorded and the simulation advances successively through events. Periods of inactivity are ignored as the simulator skips from event to event. System characteristics, such as the current system state, the simulation time, and the list of events scheduled to occur, are monitored internally in the simulation software. The following example illustrates the workings of a discrete-event simulator.

> *The first entity arrival is scheduled for time (t) = 1. The simulator moves to t = 1 and Entity 1 is added to the system, seizing Resource A. Entity 1's end of service on Resource A is scheduled for t = 6. The arrival of Entity 2 is scheduled for t = 4. The simulation moves to the next scheduled event at t = 4. Entity 2 is added to the queue for Resource A. The arrival of Entity 3 is scheduled for t = 12. At t = 6, Entity 1 completes service on Resource A and exits the system. Simultaneously, Entity 2 is removed from the queue and begins service on Resource A. Entity 2's end of service is scheduled for t = 10...*

The simulation continues, using the next-event time advance approach until the model has run for the prescribed time. The simulator then outputs a report detailing system performance. The performance measures of interest in simulation are identical to those in queuing analysis (average time in system, average number in queue, resource utilization, etc.) described earlier. However, in simulation, averages and standard deviations of these measures are provided. This requires post-processing of simulation data to get an idea of the variation around these performance statistics.

SIMULATION INPUTS AND OUTPUTS

The inputs that drive the simulation are critical to the modeling effort. Among the most important inputs to a simulation are the probability distributions used for arrival and service patterns, the initial conditions of the simulation and the run length and number of replications of the simulation.

Input Distributions

Selecting the correct statistical distributions for the time between entity arrivals and service times is an important part of developing an accurate simulation model. When fitting data to a distribution, be sure the sample size is large enough that it will provide a good idea about process variation. Once data are in hand, use an input analyzer from the simulation software, or statistical software like MINITAB, to select the statistical distribution that best describes the data. For instance, length-of-stay data might be better described by a lognormal distribution than the standard exponential distribution used in many queuing models.

Initial Simulation Conditions

Another important aspect of simulation analysis is ensuring that any "start-up bias" in the model is eliminated. When a simulation model begins with all queues and resources empty and idle, the resulting output data may be biased, if this does not reflect the actual conditions in the system being simulated. In a busy ED, for instance, it is extremely rare that all servers (beds, nurses, doctors) are idle. For this reason, it is important to select accurate initial conditions to the simulation that reflect the status of the system. Conversely, when simulating a clinic that is not open 24 hours a day, starting empty and idle may accurately reflect conditions at the time the clinic opens.

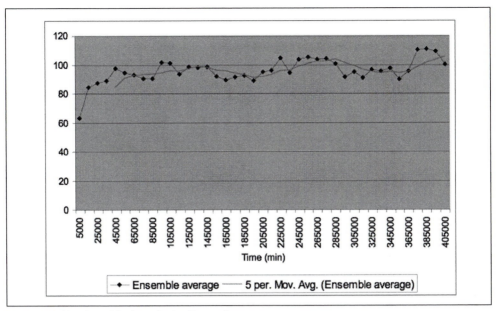

Figure 8-1: Number of Patients in the System[3]

For example, Figure 8-1 shows the number of patients in a hospital over time. There is an obvious start-up bias, as the simulation was started empty and idle. Occupancy begins to stabilize (although variation still exists) around time 35,000. Therefore, in order to reduce start-up bias, the simulation statistics should be collected only from time 35,000 and on.

Some simulation practitioners consider the practice of discarding observations to be wasteful. In this case, instead of discarding observations from time 0 to 35,000, the user might wish to pre-load the simulation with a steady-state expectation of entities in the system. In Figure 8-1, the steady-state expectation might be around 90–100 entities in the system. It is important in this case to keep track of time-of-day or day-of-week effects for system occupancy. For further insight into this subject, Law and Kelton[4] discuss initializing simulation models.

Determining Simulation Run Length

There are no definitive "right" or "wrong" simulation run lengths. The correct run length is a function of what the user would like to know about the system being analyzed. For example, if a practitioner is simulating a healthcare clinic, which closes at the end of each workday, it may be entirely reasonable to start the simulation empty and idle and use a simulated run length of eight hours.

On the other hand, if the practitioner is concerned about long-run system behaviors, such as the average number of ED patients seen per day under a given capacity, the simulation can be run for weeks or months to obtain steady-state estimates. In this case, it might not make sense to start the simulation empty and idle because of the problems with bias in early observations.

Replicating Simulations

Although a simulation will provide the user with estimates of system performance measures, it is important that the practitioner perform multiple independent replications of the simulation. Because simulation does not provide analytical solutions, the outputs of a simulation are random variables, subject to variation. As a result, multiple independent replications of a simulation allow the analyst to quantify variability and get a better estimate of true process means. There are a number of methods available to ensure independently replicated simulations. (For more information, see Banks et al.[5])

Simulation Outputs

Once multiple independent replications of a simulation are complete, the simulation package will output a report detailing system performance over the simulated time interval. When investigating specific performance measures of interest from multiple replications of a simulation, it can be useful to build **confidence intervals** on the data. Confidence intervals give a $(100 - a)\%$ confidence estimate that the mean of a process falls within the interval.

Consider the example of patient wait times to use an imaging machine in a clinic. Management is curious about the effect on wait times of adding an additional machine. The output waiting times after 10 independent replications of the proposed system are shown in Table 8-1.

Table 8-1: Wait Times for an Imaging Machine

Replication	Patient Wait Time (min)
1	5.2
2	4.3
3	6.8
4	7.1
5	3.8
6	4.5
7	5.1
8	2.9
9	5.6
10	6.0

In order to get an estimate of the mean that accounts for the observed variability, the analyst can now construct 95% ($a = 0.05$) confidence intervals using the following formula:

$$\overline{X}(n) \pm t_{n-1, 1-a/2} \sqrt{\frac{s^2(n)}{n}}$$

Where $\overline{x}(n)$ denotes the observed process average, $t_{n-1, 1-a/2}$ is found using a t-table, $s^2(n)$ denotes the observed process variance, and n denotes the number of observations. Under the observed data, the 95% confidence intervals were calculated as follows:

$$5.13 \pm t_{9,1-0.025}\sqrt{\frac{1.72}{10}} \Rightarrow 5.13 \pm (2.262)\sqrt{0.172} \Rightarrow 5.13 \pm 0.94$$

Therefore, we can say that we are 95% confident that the average patient wait time falls in the following interval [4.2, 6.1]. Although higher confidence might be desired, it is important to understand that as the alpha-level decreases (and confidence increases), confidence intervals become larger, and estimating performance statistics becomes more difficult.

Confidence intervals can also be used to compare multiple systems. In the previous example, if the analyst was interested in seeing whether a significant improvement in wait times had been made, confidence intervals from the simulated system could be compared to the 'as-is' observed wait times. If the observed 'as-is' mean wait time is within the bounds of the confidence interval for the simulated system, no significant difference between the two systems exists. For more information of system comparison, see Law and Kelton.[4]

Animation

Although not critical to a simulation model, many consider animation a benefit of using simulation. Many animation packages allow the user to import computer-aided design (CAD) objects and animate entities moving through a virtual environment. The main use of animation is to provide a viewer of the simulation with a representation of operations in the simulated system. An animated simulation will allow users to watch entities accumulate in queues, seize resources and travel through the system. While much of this information can be realized by examining output data, animation may help to impress some clients. Animation can also be used to create real-time dashboards to track performance statistics of interest.

SIMULATION PACKAGES

Unlike queuing, simulation packages are routinely quite expensive with an initial cost and annual organizational licensing costs. However, the benefits of flexibility and capabilities available in many commercial packages may offset the cost depending on application and usage. MedModel (ProModel)[6] is a simulation package designed specifically for healthcare applications. Like most modern simulation packages, it is module-based and requires little to no actual coding. Instead, modules are dragged and dropped into the simulation workspace, allowing the user to then customize the program with input data. Other quality simulation packages include ARENA (Rockwell Software),[7] AutoMod (Applied Material),[8] and SIMUL8 (SIMUL8 Corporation).[9]

ADDITIONAL SIMULATION RESOURCES

Jun et al.[10] provide a survey of more than 100 papers in the healthcare industry that use simulation to solve problems ranging, from staffing and scheduling to patient flow design and facility capacitating. For further information on simulation, a recommended text is Banks et al.[5] Their text comprehensively covers the simulation from the early developments in simulation software to applied statistics for comparing simulation designs. Also, Law and Kelton[4] cover the simulation modeling process in detail with

FORTRAN programming examples. While the FORTRAN coding may not be of interest to some readers, there are excellent discussions on the topics of probability distributions, verification and validation, and output analysis that are relevant for all simulation modelers. Some simulation languages such as ARENA (Rockwell Software)[7] have associated textbooks that are useful in introducing readers to the simulation process and the ins and outs of that specific language.

VERIFICATION AND VALIDATION

Model verification and validation are critical components to building both queuing and simulation models. **Verification** is the act of making sure that the model operates the way it is intended. **Validation** is the act of confirming that the model's system performance measure estimates accurately reflect real-world system performance. Verifying and validating a model is a critical step in the modeling process. If the model cannot be verified and validated, the model should not be used, and a different model should be considered.

Verification and validation in queuing are fairly simple. To verify the queuing model, make sure that both arrival and service time distributions match collected data, that model inputs are in the same time units, that the number of servers (c) assumed is accurate, according to the real world system, and, if calculations are done in a spreadsheet and not with software, that the formula calculations are correct. If you are modeling a queuing network, make sure that the arrival rates to each area of the network accurately portray the real system. To validate the queuing model, simply compare the model's performance measures estimates discussed earlier with data collected of the actual performance measures.

Verification and validation in a simulation model are more involved. Verification includes debugging the simulation coding and making sure all entities that flow through the model were conceptualized in the model formulation stage. While this task is simple in theory, verification of large-scale simulation models can be a time-consuming job. Animation can also be used in the verification stage. As the model runs, watch the entities build in queues, transfer among nodes and be serviced. As this is occurring, ask yourself if it mirrors what would be expected. Are huge queues being amassed at a certain area? Are entities mysteriously disappearing from the simulation? If any obvious problems exist, they must be addressed before moving on.

When conducting simulation modeling, it is important to validate the model by comparing performance statistics from a baseline simulation (using 'as-is' conditions) before experimenting with capacity or process changes. Observations from simulations can be compared with actual data using statistical hypothesis testing.

For example, consider a simulation in a clinic that serves walk-in patients. It has been observed from historical clinical data that the average patient who arrives to the clinic must wait 14 minutes before a doctor can treat him/her. After building a simulation model of the clinic and running ten replications, the simulation analyst observes the average simulated wait times shown in Table 8-2.

Table 8-2: Average Wait Times—Clinic Simulation with Ten Replications

Replication	Patient Wait Time (min)
1	13.6
2	15.7
3	12.9
4	12.2
5	13.4
6	11.9
7	12.7
8	14.5
9	15.0
10	12.1

The analyst can now use a t-test[11] to compare differences in the simulated output with the actual clinic data as follows. Assume the analyst chooses an alpha level of 0.05 in order to achieve 95% (1–alpha) confidence in the conclusions. The initial hypothesis (H_0) is that the average wait time W_q equals 14 minutes and the alternate hypothesis (H_1) is that W_q is not 14 minutes.

H_0: W_q = 14 min

H_1: $W_q \neq$ 14 min

The observed mean from the simulations ($\bar{Y}$) is equal to 13.4. The observed standard deviation (S) equals 1.3. The mean was calculated from 10 replications (n=10). Therefore, the test statistic is calculated as follows:

$$t_0 = \frac{\bar{Y} - \mu_0}{S/\sqrt{n}} = \frac{13.4 - 14}{1.3/\sqrt{10}} = -1.46$$

We can reject our null hypothesis (H_0) if $|t_0| > t_{a/2,n-1}$. From a t-table, we see that $t_{0.025,9}$ = 2.26. Since 1.46 < 2.26, we cannot reject H_0, and we therefore conclude that there is no significant difference in performance between the simulation and the real system. Now we can move on to experiment with changes to the system in order to see the effects on clinic performance.

SUMMARY

Queuing and simulation modeling are very powerful tools that can help healthcare organizations make educated decisions on capacity levels and estimate delays in customer service, such as waiting. This chapter presents an applied approach to queuing and simulation modeling. Using the information in this chapter, the reader can understand the different common types of queuing systems, why queues form, and when to use queuing or simulation modeling. System performance measures are presented to provide the reader with guidelines for evaluating operations.

The four-step modeling process presented here is applicable to any modeling effort and provides the reader with a structured approach for problem solving. Queuing formulae and analytical results are presented for many queue types that are common in a healthcare setting. Additionally, the discrete-event computer simulation process is introduced to give the reader a high-level view of system simulation and an understanding of the essential simulation inputs. Lastly, this chapter discusses model verification and validation techniques to ensure the model accurately represents real-world behaviors. Throughout the chapter, additional resources are provided such as software packages, books, and journal articles are recommended as supplemental information to enhance the reader's understanding of these subjects.

References

1. Kirtland A, Lockwood J, Poisker K, Stamp L, Wolfe P. Simulating an emergency department "Is as much fun as…" In Alexopoulos C, Kang K, Lilegdon WR, Goldsman D (eds). *Proceedings of the 1995 Winter Simulation Conference.* 1995; 1039-1042.
2. Harper PR, Shahani AK. Modeling for the planning and management of bed capacities in hospitals. *Journal of the Operational Research Society.* 2002;53:11-18.
3. Cochran JK, Bharti A. Stochastic bed balancing of an obstetrics hospital. *Health Care Management Science.* 2006; 9(1):31-45.
4. Law AM, Kelton WD. *Simulation Modeling and Analysis.* New York: McGraw-Hill; 2000.
5. Banks J, Carson JS, Nelson BL, Nicol DM. *Discrete-Event System Simulation.* Prentice Hall; 2000.
6. ProModel. MedModel. http://www.promodel.com/products/medmodel/.
7. Rockwell Software. Arena. http://www.arenasimulation.com/.
8. Applied Material. AutoMod software. www.brookssoftware.com.
9. SIMUL8 Corporation. SIMUL8. http://www.simul8.com/.
10. Jun JB, Jacobson SH, Swisher JR. Applications of discrete-event simulation in healthcare clinics: A survey. *Journal of the Operational Research Society.* 199; (50):109-123.
11. Montgomery DC, Runger GC, Hubele NF. *Engineering Statistics.* New York: John Wiley & Sons; 2006.

CHAPTER 9

Productivity Management

John Hansmann

> *"Productivity is being able to do things that you were never able to do before."*
>
> — Franz Kafka

INTRODUCTION

The concepts of **productivity** and **productivity management** have been around for many years. Although the constructs have not significantly changed over time, some of the measurements have. Productivity measures have historically centered on the hospital, and primarily on labor consumption. However, as hospitals have grown or merged into healthcare delivery systems, including physician operations and health plans, productivity measures have changed as well. In this chapter, we first explore traditional productivity measurement approaches, then discuss new twists to traditional monitoring/measurement.

HEALTHCARE ENVIRONMENT

The current healthcare environment is ever changing, and it appears this change will continue for the foreseeable future. The population is aging, and because most Americans use more healthcare as they get older, more healthcare resources will be consumed in the future. Today, healthcare spending represents 16% of the gross domestic product (GDP) and is estimated to reach 20% in the next decade. Currently, 47 million Americans do not have healthcare insurance. That number increases by approximately 300,000 individuals for every one percent increase in healthcare costs. The issue of quality in healthcare has been evaluated and challenged, especially since 1999, when the Institute of Medicine released the report, *To Err is Human*,[1] which stated that between 44,000 and 98,000 people die each year due to medical errors. Genomics, regenerative medicine and consumerism will direct how healthcare is delivered in the future. All of this is happening at the same time that Medicare, Medicaid and commercial insurance companies are attempting to reduce their costs, which typically means reduced revenue for healthcare organizations.

It is very clear that the American healthcare delivery system is being challenged in ways it has not been in the past. Although many of the aforementioned issues are somewhat out of the control of healthcare organizations, those organizations do control how they manage the resources used to provide care. In managing change, specifically the immense cost pressures placed on the system, a focus on productivity and productivity management will have a major impact on the cost of operations of these healthcare organizations. Management engineers have traditionally been the productivity experts for their healthcare organizations. It is time again for MEs to act as advocates and lead the change for improving productivity in the healthcare system.

TRADITIONAL PRODUCTIVITY MONITORING

A fundamental aspect of any ME's skill set is the understanding of productivity and productivity management concepts.[2] By understanding these concepts, an ME can easily apply the concepts of work measurement, work simplification, operations analysis, process improvement, staffing analysis and future workforce planning. All are analytical concepts whose outcome is intended to improve the use of labor resources in an organization.

What Is Productivity?

Productivity is the measure of output to input of a system. Different industries use different measures or indicators for productivity. The healthcare industry typically uses the number of patients receiving care/services (the number of patients each day for whom care was provided—patient days, procedures performed on patients, or patient visits) as a measure of output from the system. The input typically referenced is either the cost or the number of labor hours expended to process or take care of the patients. A ratio of dollars or hours per number of patients processed (or unit of measure) is calculated. Historically, organizations used only labor hours expended as the primary input variable to the calculation. However, as the cost of care has become an issue, dollars per unit of measure have become the primary indicator, with the hour per unit of measure indicator becoming a secondary measure; however, when used in conjunction with the dollars per unit of measure, an organization can understand a lot about its labor resources.

Inputs and Outputs of a Productivity System

The two components of the ratio—the inputs and outputs of a productivity system—need further examination. The typical inputs, labor dollars/hours, require additional understanding. Two types of labor dollars/hours are reported in the healthcare industry—productive and total. Productive dollars/hours are defined as those dollars/hours used to perform patient processes. These include regular, overtime, and premium dollars/hours (e.g., for shift differential, on call and call back), time when employees are actually at work. Total dollars/hours include productive dollars/hours plus nonproductive dollars/hours paid for time off, such as vacation, holiday, and illness (termed *personal time off* or PTO.)

Productive dollars/hours can be further broken down into *fixed* and *variable* components. Positions that in general fluctuate with workload volume can be considered variable. Typically this category would include nurses, respiratory therapists, radiology technologists and others who are directly involved in the performance of the primary unit of measure for the department. Fixed positions, on the other hand, which usually support the performance of the direct caregivers, typically include managers and unit secretaries. (The same can be said for ancillary or support departments as well.)

Some organizations even separate fixed positions into *direct* and *indirect* positions. Direct fixed time is time involved in directly supporting the main operation of the area, such as a manager or unit secretary. Indirect fixed time is time used in preparing for the future, such as time used for employee orientation, training/education and staff meetings. Although most organizations do not separate to this level, it seems fairly obvious that if an organization has the information systems to allow this level of detail, the process can be better understood.

In theory, with appropriate training, any employee can be assigned to perform any required task, a scenario in which managers and organizations have high control over productive dollars/hours. At the same time, however, managers and organizations have little control over nonproductive, or PTO, dollars/hours. Many organizations have policies in place that give incentives to employees to use their PTO time ("use it or lose it," with maximum carryover from one year to the next, etc.). Because of the control over productive dollars/hours, organizations typically use productive dollars/hours per unit of measure to track productivity. It is important to track total dollars/hours per unit of measure because of the impact on the overall operating expense for the organization, but only as a secondary indicator.

The other half of the productivity ratio is the output, or volume of patients treated. A different unit of measure is typically used for each department. The unit of measure is determined by the volume indicator that best identifies, or accounts for the primary function of the department. For nursing units, the unit of measure generally used is patient days, which is a count of the number of patients receiving care each day. Emergency departments track the number of patient visits, whereas laboratories track the number of patient tests.

Observation and short-stay patients are usually included in the inpatient day counts, but their measurement may be modified by the actual amount of time spent in the area. For example, a patient staying on a unit only 12 hours may be counted as half a patient day (12 hours divided by 24 hours). In addition, some organizations use their inpatient acuity system, or case mix index to weight or adjust their patient counts based on acuity or resource intensiveness in each case. In general, inpatient units and many other departments use a simple count of the number of patients cared for as the unit of measure. The appendix shows the typical units of measure used in each department in a healthcare organization.

Relative Value Unit

Another commonly used department unit of measure is the relative value unit (RVU). **Relative value units** are a weighted volume unit, typically used in ancillary and other departments in which traditional volume counts vary dramatically in length, complexity or intensity of service provided. For example, the typical unit of measure used in a radiology department is procedures. But relative value is seen in the fact that one procedure may not require the same amount of resources as another; for example, it typically requires approximately 15 minutes to complete a simple x-ray procedure (chest, ankle, etc.), whereas a period of 60 minutes or more is required to perform an angiography procedure. Yet each is counted as one procedure. In order to indicate a difference in value, the RVU system uses a weighting multiplier against each procedure count to determine the actual volume count for each procedure. The weighting multiplier is generally related to the time factor involved in completing the procedure. An example of a few RVU values used in a radiology department is provided in Table 9-1.

General Units of Measure

In addition to department-specific units of measure, general units of measure are also calculated. Admissions, discharges, patient days and beds are typically modified to include inpatient and outpatient activity, but because the dimensions of an inpatient day are much different than those of an outpatient visit, an adjustment calculation is performed. The calculation is based purely on financial measurement, and accounts for outpatient activity in inpatient terms. Total revenue for the organization is divided by inpatient revenue; the quotient is multiplied by the statistic being adjusted to calculate an adjusted "statistic." Inpatient admissions, discharges and patient days are used to calculate adjusted admissions, discharges and patient days, respectively. The adjusted admission and discharge statistics provide an estimate of an overall case count for the organization. In essence, when used in the calculation of expense per adjusted admission (or discharge), an estimated cost per case is developed. For a department, the result can be interpreted as the amount of the overall cost per case attributable to the department. When used in conjunction with the labor expense per unit of measure, the estimated cost per case indicator identifies a measure for utilization. For example, a productivity report that shows a laboratory that has a low cost per test but a high cost per adjusted admission indicates that a large number of laboratory tests are being performed per patient.

Adjusted patient days are an estimation of the total number of patients receiving inpatient care. The volume of outpatient visits is translated into an estimated number of inpatients using the financial adjustment previously discussed. Hundreds of thousands of outpatient visits become the equivalent of only a few thousand inpatient days. That is appropriate because, as is easily seen, it would take many blood tests and chest x-rays to equate to the amount of work required to take care of an inpatient.

Another general statistic, adjusted occupied beds, is calculated by dividing adjusted patient days by the number of calendar days in the calculation period. **Adjusted occupied beds** (AOBs) are interpreted as the total number of beds that would be occupied if all patient activity occurred in inpatient beds. In general, all of the adjusted statistics assume that high volume outpatient activity, when modified by the charge ratio (total revenue/ inpatient revenue), consumes an equivalent amount of resources compared with those used in inpatient care. Although these measures provide a sense of the organization's level of productivity and busyness, they are "ballpark" indicators at best.

In addition to the general statistics of adjusted admission, patient days and occupied beds, many organizations also now measure salary expense per net revenue and supply expense per net revenue. Such measures originated in the for-profit world of healthcare,

Table 9-1: RVU Codes

Code #	Description	RVU
1	Facial bones <3 views	69
2	Facial bones 3+ CP	76
3	Digital screen mammography	70
4	Sinuses 3+ views CP	69
5	Skull < 4 views	69
6	Skull 4+ views CP	69
7	TM joints-bilateral	69
8	Chest 1 view, frontal	52
9	Chest 2 views, front & lateral	56
10	Chest 2 views w/oblique	61
11	Spine entire, AP an lateral	81
12	Spine cerv 1 view	69
13	Spine lumbar 1 view	66
14	Spine thoracic 1 view	66
15	Spine thoracolumbar 1 view	66
16	Cerv spine, 2 or 3 views	66
17	Cerv spine 4+ views	76
18	Cerv spine CP oblique/flex	86
19	Thoracic spine 3 views	69
20	T-L spine, AP & lateral views	66
21	T-L spine scolio sup/ert	81
22	Lumbosacral spine 2-3 views	63
23	Lumbosacral spine comp & oblique	72
24	Lumbosacral spine CP w/bend	96
25	L-S spine bend only >=4 views	81
26	Pelvis 1 or 2 views	61
27	Pelvis CP min 3 views	66
28	Shoulder 1 view	61
29	Shoulder CP min 2 views	63
30	AC joints bilateral	72
31	Elbow AP & lateral views	61
32	Elbow 3+ views	63
33	Forearm 2 views	61
34	Upper ext infant 2+ views	76
35	Wrist 2 views	61
36	Wrist 3+ views	61
37	Hand 2 views	59
38	Hand 3+ views	61
39	Finger(s) 2+ views	59
40	Hip unilateral 1 view	72

and it is appropriate that it has not been limited to just that sector. All healthcare providers should be concerned about how much of their revenue is consumed by labor and supply expenses. With the bottom lines of most healthcare organizations shrinking with time, a minor shift in either of these two indicators should send a major signal to management.

The primary indicator for productivity is dollars per unit of measure. The secondary indicator, hours per unit of measure, can actually lead to incorrect conclusions if not used in conjunction with the primary indicator. If an organization decides to change its skill mix in an area in which additional, lower paid employees are hired, the hours per unit of measure may actually increase. But if this results in fewer dollars per unit of measure, the change is the right one to make (from a financial perspective). The reverse is also true; fewer higher paid staff can improve the hours per unit of measure indicator but have a negative impact on the dollars per unit of measure indicator. It is imperative to track both indicators, but the dollars per unit of measure must be the one analyzed first. Table 9-2 summarizes the formulas described earlier.

Table 9-2: Productivity Equations

Productivity	Total Outputs ÷ Total Inputs
Adjusted patient days	(Total revenue ÷ inpatient revenue) x # of patient days
Expense per adjusted admission	Total expenses ÷ adjusted patient days
Adjusted occupied beds	Adjusted patient days ÷ # of calendar days
Salary expense per net revenue	Salary expense ÷ net revenues

Scorecard Reporting

To assist managers in tracking productivity, a scorecard or reporting mechanism needs to be developed. Using a scorecard methodology, multiple indicators can be tracked simultaneously on the same report, providing a diverse look at the state of the department or organization. For productivity monitoring, the elements of the scorecard should be productive dollars/hours per unit of measure and productive dollars/hours per adjusted admission. To expand the productivity measurement system slightly, but to allow a greater sense of operations, a supply cost per unit of measure should also be included. For most organizations, labor and supply expenses account for most of the total direct expenses. Monitoring both on the same scorecard would provide the department or organization with a fairly comprehensive view of operations. To round out the scorecard, quality indicators, such as patient satisfaction and/or employee satisfaction, should also be tracked.

Productivity Index

When tracking productivity, an additional measure that is typically reported is a productivity index or percentage of productivity. The productivity index identifies how well a department is operating relative to a target value. The target value can be determined with many different approaches, such as detailed staffing/operations analysis, historical performance ratios, external comparisons (benchmarking) or negotiation. The actual productivity performance, dollars per unit of measure for a specific period, is compared with the target ratio. If the actual performance indicator is less than the target, productivity index is greater than 1 (or greater than 100%). If the actual performance indicator is greater than the target, the productivity index is less than 1 (or less than 100%). A realistic productivity performance index range would be 0.95 to 1.05 (95% to 105% productivity). When the target value is equal to the maximum capacity of the system, such as using the total number of hours possible in a specific period, the maximum productivity index would be 1 (100%), with the expected range being less.

Studying the trend of scorecard indicators over time allows an organization to determine if a specific area of the organization is becoming more or less productive (using more or fewer dollars/hours to treat the same number of patients). Organizations are said to be becoming more productive when they are using fewer dollars/hours to treat the same number of patients compared with that ratio during a previous period. These comparisons also allow managers to use information to better manage their areas and the organization's resources.

Links to Budgeting Systems

The final aspect of a well-performing productivity management system is providing a formal link to the organization's budgeting system, which monitors overall expenditures for the organization. The productivity management system is the primary monitoring device to track labor resources in an organization. In most healthcare organizations, labor expenses equal approximately 50% of total expenses. Providing a formal link, with which labor productivity data from the productivity management system are shared with the budget system and reported on common reports, will allow management to see how its plan (budget) was actually implemented (productivity management). A better and more realistic labor budget can be developed for future years by monitoring and controlling current labor expenses with the productivity management system. Using this information year after year creates an upward-spiraling process that results in better labor expense control and a realistic understanding of the true labor costs of the organization. A well-functioning productivity management system can lead to a more effective budgeting system.

PRODUCTIVITY REPORTING AND USES

The primary use of a productivity monitoring system is to track labor usage throughout the organization. Departments that are more productive, as well as those that are becoming less productive, are known. To really use the information effectively, the monitoring system needs to be elevated to a productivity management system. When that occurs, the uses for the information dramatically increase.

Under a productivity management system philosophy, the department or organization becomes very proactive in using the productivity information. Six main uses of the information are shown in Table 9-3.

Table 9-3: Uses of Productivity Information

#	Uses of Productivity Information
1	Cost control and savings identification
2	Management/tracking appropriate labor usage
3	Staffing level determination (resource allocation)
4	Identification of productivity improvement ideas
5	Future workforce determination
6	Development of appropriate service levels

The first three uses shown in the table are related by the desire to control labor expenses and appropriately allocate labor resources. The productivity monitoring system identifies those departments that use too many resources for the amount of work they are performing. Based on the information gathered, the managers of the identified areas have an obligation and responsibility to more appropriately assign resources to accomplish the required tasks, which means adjusting staffing levels. Managers can become more creative with staffing assignments and allocation of resources when they have good productivity information to use.

Productivity management reports include data that are important to an organization to measure. When comparing reports across organizations, many common elements exist. Every department or reporting unit generally has its own report that includes both data and graphical elements. Departments are typically grouped into a common organizational structure reporting to an administrative officer (titles such as vice president, operations officer, etc.). Usually a roll-up report is provided for each administrative officer, as well as a roll-up summary for the entire organization. Examples of typical reports along with a brief explanation are provided in the next sections.

Departmental Reporting—Productive Salary

Figure 9-1 provides a simple yet very useful and powerful view of a department's productivity performance. The most useful graphs show data over time, such as the monthly data seen in this example. The graph tracks actual productive salary dollars per patient day (diamond symbol), target (or expected) performance (square symbol), the acceptable range of performance using a "control chart like" concept of upper and lower limits (dashes), benchmark or "best practice" comparator (squares) and actual trendline (solid line.)

The actual performance is calculated by dividing the actual productive salary dollars by the number of patient days for each time period represented. The target value can be set in many different ways, but the practice most commonly seen is to equate budget to target, which reinforces the message that a department needs to run on budget. And by measuring on a cost per unit basis, the argument that increased volume caused a budget overage is minimized. The upper and lower limits are set in two ways; using a reasonable variance limit ($\pm$ 5 percent in this case), or using actual control chart methodology and calculating historical variation. The benchmark or "best practice" comparator is typically provided as a goal indicator that the department is to strive for

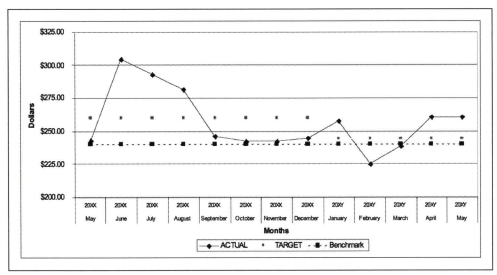

Figure 9-1: Productive Salary Dollars per Patient Day

and achieve over time. The trendline shows the overall direction of the department's actual productivity performance during the time period reported.

The power of this report is that, in a glance, the department manager can see how well the department has been performing on a productive salary per patient day basis over time. In the case of the example shown, the department has been performing better over time, yet its performance in the new year seems to be a little less productive than that shown for the end of the previous year. To find out more details, the department manager should look at the associated department report. The same type of graph can be developed for the productive hours per unit of measure indicators as well.

Departmental Reporting—Productivity Management

Figure 9-2 provides the data detail used to create the department productivity graph, plus more. Typically the department report will include actual and budget data for such key elements as workload volume, productive dollars and corresponding productive dollars per unit of measure indicator for each reporting time period. Variance data are provided to show deviation from budget or expectations. Month-to-date and year-to-date data are provided, and now more prevalent than before is the addition of last "x" time periods of data (12 previous months in the example provided) used to show a contiguous time period of data. Additional data elements may be provided, such as overtime usage and 6-month forecast (expected performance for the next 6 months based on forecasted volume, budget and workload indicators), shown in this example. Healthcare organizations with more sophisticated systems will report data to the individual job code or general ledger account levels. Some very large departments with multiple functional sections may develop a department report for each section. But the importance of this report is the detail provided to management to demonstrate how effective it is using its resources, areas of strength and where there are opportunities for improvement. Similar to the graph in Figure 9-1, this report can be developed for hours per unit of measure indicators as well.

MONTH	YR	WORKLOAD ACTUAL	WORKLOAD FORCST	WORKLOAD %VAR	WORKED $$$ ACTUAL	WORKED $$$ PLANNED	WORKED $$$ %VAR	Paid $$$ ACTUAL	Paid $$$ BUDGET	Paid $$$ %VAR	BENFT & EDUC %	WRK $$$/WORKLOAD ACTUAL	WRK $$$/WORKLOAD TARGET	WRK $$$/WORKLOAD %VAR	PD $$$/WORKLOAD ACTUAL	PD $$$/WORKLOAD TARGET	PD $$$/WORKLOAD %VAR	%UTLZ	LL	UL	Bench mark
May	20XX	797	792	0.63%	$193,575	$201,451	3.91%	$211,999	$223,834	5.58%	8.4%	$242.88	$260.00	6.58%	$265.24	286.00	7.26%	107.0%	247.00	273	$240.00
June	20XX	622	731	-14.91%	$189,386	$194,937	2.85%	$211,226	$216,619	2.49%	10.4%	$304.48	$280.00	-17.11%	$339.59	286.00	-18.74%	85.4%	247.00	273	$240.00
July	20XX	610	772	-20.98%	$178,745	$201,451	11.27%	$214,623	$223,834	4.12%	16.5%	$293.02	$260.00	-12.70%	$351.84	286.00	-23.02%	83.3%	247.00	273	$240.00
August	20XX	621	772	-19.58%	$174,922	$201,451	13.17%	$213,067	$223,834	4.81%	17.9%	$281.68	$260.00	-8.34%	$343.09	286.00	-19.96%	92.3%	247.00	273	$240.00
September	20XX	619	726	-14.74%	$152,436	$194,997	21.83%	$178,555	$216,619	17.57%	14.6%	$246.26	$260.00	5.28%	$288.46	286.00	-0.86%	105.6%	247.00	273	$240.00
October	20XX	747	812	-8.00%	$180,863	$201,451	10.22%	$208,866	$223,834	6.69%	13.4%	$242.12	$260.00	6.88%	$279.61	286.00	2.24%	107.4%	247.00	273	$240.00
November	20XX	726	761	-4.60%	$175,856	$194,937	9.83%	$197,843	$216,619	8.67%	11.2%	$242.20	$260.00	6.85%	$272.65	286.00	4.67%	105.3%	247.00	273	$240.00
December	20XX	725	740	-2.03%	$177,363	$201,451	11.96%	$202,003	$223,834	9.75%	12.2%	$244.64	$260.00	5.91%	$278.63	286.00	2.58%	94.7%	247.00	273	$240.00
January	20XY	720	777	-7.34%	$185,745	$184,870	-0.47%	$204,398	$205,412	0.49%	9.1%	$257.98	$244.40	-5.56%	$283.88	273.60	-3.01%	94.7%	232.18	256.62	$240.00
February	20XY	750	697	7.60%	$168,605	$166,982	-0.97%	$186,285	$185,536	-0.40%	9.5%	$224.81	$244.40	8.02%	$248.38	273.60	9.88%	108.7%	232.18	256.62	$240.00
March	20XY	730	731	-0.78%	$186,252	$184,870	-0.78%	$209,050	$205,412	-1.77%	10.9%	$255.78	$244.40	2.39%	$268.01	273.60	2.75%	102.4%	232.18	256.62	$240.00
April	20XY	663	697	-5.02%	$172,557	$184,870	3.56%	$199,053	$198,790	-0.13%	13.3%	$260.63	$244.40	-6.64%	$300.69	273.60	-9.10%	93.8%	232.18	256.62	$240.00
May	20XY	658	743	-11.44%	$171,422	$184,870	7.27%	$207,354	$205,412	-0.90%	17.3%	$260.52	$244.40	-6.60%	$314.98	273.60	-14.39%	93.0%	232.18	256.62	$240.00
Y-T-D May	20XY	3570	3645	-2.06%	$884,562	$900,505	1.77%	$1,006,045	$1,000,561	-0.55%	12.1%	$247.78	244.40	-1.38%	$281.81	275.60	-2.22%	98.6%			
LY-T-D May	20XX	3911	3887	0.62%	$951,206	$981,268	3.00%	$1,065,171	$1,060,297	-0.30%	10.7%	$243.21	260.00	6.46%	$272.35	286.00	4.77%	106.9%			
LST 12 P May	20XY	8240	8959	-8.03%	$2,114,112	$2,291,179	7.73%	$2,432,317	$2,485,734	4.46%	13.1%	$256.57	255.30	-1.23%	$280.18	281.58	-4.83%	93.0%			

OVERTIME DOLLARS / **OVERTIME PERCENT**

	OVERTIME DOLLARS	OVERTIME PERCENT
CURRENT	$3,081	1.80%
Y-T-D	$22,918	2.39%
LAST 12 PERIODS	$31,108	1.47%

WORKED VARIANCE / **PAID VARIANCE**

	WORKED VARIANCE	PAID VARIANCE
	$(10,607)	$(25,909)
	$(312,054)	$(32,153)
	$(525,272)	$(112,098)

IMPACT OF VARIANCE:
POSITIVE - UNDER TARGET $$$
NEGATIVE - OVER TARGET $$$

6 MONTH FORECAST

MONTH	WORKLOAD FORECAST	YEAR	WORKED $$$ REQD	WORKED $$$ PLANNED	%VAR	PAID $$$ REQD	PAID $$$ BUDGET	%VAR	WRK $$$/WORKLOAD ACTUAL	TARGET	PLANNED	PD $$$/WORKLOAD TARGET	BUDGET
June	720	20XY	$175,968	$178,911	1.65%	$198,432	$198,790	0.18%	$248.49	$244.40	$244.40	$275.60	$276.10
July	708	20XY	$173,035	$184,870	6.40%	$195,125	$205,412	5.01%	$281.12	$244.40	$244.40	$275.60	$290.13
August	720	20XY	$175,968	$184,870	4.82%	$198,432	$205,412	3.40%	$256.76	$244.40	$244.40	$275.60	$285.29
September	697	20XY	$170,347	$178,911	4.79%	$192,093	$198,790	3.37%	$256.69	$244.40	$244.40	$275.60	$285.21
October	788	20XY	$192,587	$184,870	-4.17%	$217,173	$205,412	-5.73%	$231.61	$244.40	$244.40	$275.60	$260.67
November	771	20XY	$188,432	$178,911	-5.32%	$212,488	$198,790	-6.89%	$232.05	$244.40	$244.40	$275.60	$257.83

Figure 9-2: Productivity Management—Department Report

Administrative Roll-Up Report

Figure 9-3 provides a summary report to each administrative officer for all their reporting departments. Each line item represents a department summary brought forward from the department reports, which typically includes actual and budget data for such key elements as workload volume, productive dollars and corresponding productive dollars per unit of measure indicator for each reporting time period. Month-to-date and year-to-date data are provided, and in some cases the last "x" time periods of data (12 previous months in the example provided) are used to show a contiguous time period of data. Additional data elements may be provided, such as percent productivity utilization and exceptions columns (which are flagged if a department's performance is outside the expected variance range) as shown in this example. The value of this report is that it provides the administrative officer a high level summary of each of the direct report departments. If further detail is required, the administrative officer can refer to the department report.

Facility Roll-Up Report

Figure 9-4 provides a summary report for the overall facility/organization. Each line item represents an administrative officer summary brought forward from the VP summary reports. As with the other summary reports, this report typically includes actual and budget data for such key elements as productive dollars and hours/full time equivalents month and year-to-date. They usually do not include administrative roll-up or departmental level productivity indicators because the indicators are not additive and cannot be reported in this manner. General indicators, such as adjusted admission, patient days and occupied beds can and typically are reported on this type of a roll-up report. Obviously, the value of this report is that it provides a high level view of the entire organization. If further detail is required, the administrative summaries or department reports can be referenced.

Scorecard Report

Figure 9-5 provides a snapshot overview of six key indicators that are important for an organization to monitor. Typically organizations will monitor labor productivity, supply expense, revenue and, in many cases, quality as well as other indicators. Usually these charts are shown over a longer time period for trending purposes. The example shown provides three graphs as an expense per net revenue percent, identifying the percent of revenue spent on staff salaries, supplies and benefits (top three graphs horizontally across the page). The bottom three graphs show high level organizational productivity indicators, comparing staff salaries, supply expense and productive FTEs (full time equivalents) per AOB. The interpretation of theses graphs provides a number of interesting observations:

- As a percentage of net revenue, salary expense is declining (positive), and is due to two factors: (1) decreasing FTEs and (2) increasing revenue.
- Supply and benefit expense as a percent of net revenue is static.
- Supply expense per AOB is increasing over time, even though the percent of revenue is static. The probable cause is higher supply rate, although reduced volume could also be a contributing factor.

CST		SALARY DOLLARS						OVERTIME		PRODUCTIVITY INDICATORS													
		WORKED $$$			PAID $$$			PERCENT		WRK $$$/WORKLOAD			PERCENT UTIL		EXCEPT			PD $$$/WORKLOAD			EXCEPT		
CTR	COST CENTER NAME	CURRENT	YTD	PLAN	CURRENT	YTD	BUDGET	CURR	YTD	CURR	YTD	TARGET	CURR	YTD	C	Y	LP	CURR	YTD	TARGET	C	Y	LP
305	SURG CARDIAC	$171,422	$884,562	$900,505	$207,254	$1,006,045	$1,000,561	1.0%	1.5%	$260.52	$247.78	$244.40	93.8%	98.6%	#		11	$314.98	$281.81	$275.60	#		6
306	MED/CARDIAC	$166,512	$836,955	$834,798	$188,831	$927,984	$927,553	1.0%	1.2%	$221.75	$214.75	$210.00	94.7%	97.8%	#		8	$251.47	$238.11	$225.00	#	#	9
307	MED/RESP	$176,219	$863,530	$844,272	$200,367	$957,752	$938,080	0.9%	0.7%	$212.40	$203.76	$212.40	100.0%	104.2%			7	$241.51	$225.99	$238.32		#	7
308	NEUROLOGY	$164,671	$818,645	$817,713	$184,615	$904,843	$908,571	0.4%	0.7%	$204.39	$206.55	$210.60	103.0%	102.0%			6	$229.14	$228.30	$237.60			7
309	SURG/GU	$172,180	$856,584	$821,208	$195,297	$947,183	$912,453	0.5%	0.9%	$197.25	$190.00	$190.00	96.3%	100.0%			7	$223.73	$210.10	$210.00	#		8
325	PEDIATRICS	$57,526	$298,974	$283,443	$68,243	$335,860	$314,937	0.6%	0.8%	$258.00	$219.75	$215.00	83.3%	97.8%	#		10	$306.06	$246.86	$222.50	#	#	7
335	MICU	$100,538	$521,121	$624,040	$119,683	$603,988	$693,378	0.1%	0.1%	$515.48	$525.84	$666.40	129.3%	126.7%	#	#	9	$613.64	$609.46	$725.20	#	#	10
336	SICU	$175,739	$813,477	$844,505	$201,013	$929,831	$938,339	2.1%	1.3%	$559.70	$560.28	$728.48	130.2%	130.0%	#	#	10	$640.19	$640.42	$797.50	#	#	10
337	CICU	$90,288	$459,203	$535,824	$110,535	$540,819	$595,360	0.4%	0.2%	$567.60	$551.70	$735.00	129.5%	133.2%	#	#	11	$694.88	$649.76	$816.00	#	#	9
340	EMERGENCY	$247,351	$1,176,569	$1,095,876	$284,104	$1,331,673	$1,217,640	2.5%	1.9%	$59.08	$56.28	$61.60	104.3%	109.5%		#	6	$67.86	$63.70	$67.20		#	8
420	RESPIRATORY CARE	$112,392	$562,831	$544,987	$129,812	$623,005	$605,541	1.2%	1.1%	$55.66	$55.88	$64.46	115.8%	115.4%	#	#	12	$64.29	$61.85	$70.62	#	#	11
441	PHARMACY	$192,268	$886,050	$834,021	$200,877	$929,020	$926,690	0.2%	0.1%	$15.60	$14.40	$12.30	78.8%	85.4%	#	#	9	$16.30	$15.10	$13.80	#	#	9
550	SOCIAL WORK SERVICES	$56,685	$286,635	$284,219	$64,337	$178,263	$315,799	0.0%	0.0%	$77.20	$71.40	$69.20	89.6%	96.9%	#		7	$87.62	$44.40	$78.20	#		8
	Total VP Nursing & Pat Care Ser	$1,883,790	$9,265,137	$9,265,411	$2,154,968	$10,216,266	$10,294,901																

CST		FULL TIME EQUIVALENTS						OVERTIME		PRODUCTIVITY INDICATORS													
		WORKED FTEs			PAID FTEs			PERCENT		WRK HRS/WORKLOAD			PERCENT UTIL		EXCEPT			PD HRS/WORKLOAD			EXCEPT		
CTR	COST CENTER NAME	CURRENT	YTD	PLAN	CURRENT	YTD	BUDGET	CURR	YTD	CURR	YTD	TARGET	CURR	YTD	C	Y	LP	CURR	YTD	TARGET	C	Y	LP
305	SURG CARDIAC	37.22	39.44	40.14	45.00	44.86	44.60	1.0%	1.5%	10.02	9.53	9.40	93.5%	98.6%	#		11	12.11	10.84	10.60	#		6
306	MED/CARDIAC	37.60	38.80	38.70	42.64	43.02	43.00	1.0%	1.2%	8.87	8.59	8.40	94.7%	97.8%	#		8	10.06	9.52	9.00	#	#	9
307	MED/RESP	41.45	41.70	40.77	47.13	46.25	45.30	0.9%	0.7%	8.85	8.49	8.85	100.0%	104.3%			7	10.06	9.41	9.93		#	7
308	NEUROLOGY	34.43	35.14	35.10	38.60	38.84	39.00	0.4%	0.7%	7.57	7.65	7.80	103.1%	101.9%			6	8.48	8.46	8.80			7
309	SURG/GU	38.88	39.71	38.07	44.10	43.91	42.30	0.5%	0.9%	7.89	7.60	7.60	96.3%	100.0%			7	8.95	8.41	8.40	#		8
325	PEDIATRICS	12.99	13.86	13.14	15.41	15.57	14.60	0.6%	0.8%	10.32	8.79	8.60	83.4%	97.9%	#		10	12.24	9.87	8.90	#	#	7
335	MICU	20.27	21.57	25.83	24.13	25.00	28.70	0.1%	0.1%	18.41	18.78	23.80	129.3%	126.7%	#	#	9	21.92	21.77	25.90	#	#	10
336	SICU	34.21	32.51	33.75	39.13	37.16	37.50	2.1%	1.3%	19.30	19.32	25.12	130.2%	130.0%	#	#	10	22.07	22.08	27.50	#	#	10
337	CICU	16.99	17.74	20.70	20.80	20.89	23.00	0.4%	0.2%	18.92	18.39	24.50	129.5%	133.2%	#	#	11	23.18	21.66	27.20	#	#	9
340	EMERGENCY	49.87	48.70	45.36	57.28	55.12	50.40	2.5%	1.9%	2.11	2.01	2.20	104.1%	109.4%		#	6	2.43	2.28	2.40		#	8
420	RESPIRATORY CARE	28.84	29.65	28.71	33.31	32.82	31.90	1.2%	1.1%	2.53	2.54	2.93	116.0%	115.4%	#	#	12	2.92	2.81	3.21	#	#	11
441	PHARMACY	36.18	34.23	32.22	37.80	35.89	35.80	0.2%	0.1%	0.52	0.48	0.41	78.8%	85.4%	#	#	9	0.54	0.50	0.46	#	#	9
550	SOCIAL WORK SERVICES	16.00	16.61	16.47	18.16	10.33	18.30	0.0%	0.0%	3.86	3.57	3.46	89.6%	97.0%	#		7	4.38	3.94	3.91	#		8
	Total VP Nursing & Pat Care Ser	404.93	409.66	408.96	463.49	449.66	454.40																

Figure 9-3: Productivity Management—VP Summary Report

RESPONSIBILITY ROLL UP	SALARY DOLLARS						FULL TIME EQUIVALENTS					
	WORKED $$$			PAID $$$			WORKED FTEs			PAID FTEs		
	CURRENT	YTD	PLAN	CURRENT	YTD	BUDGET	CURRENT	YTD	PLAN	CURRENT	YTD	BUDGET
VP NURSING & PT CARE SER	$1,883,790	$9,265,137	$9,265,411	$2,154,968	$10,216,266	$10,294,901	404.93	409.66	408.96	463.49	449.66	454.40
VP ANCILLARY SERVICES	$1,308,606	$6,419,524	$6,092,134	$1,394,406	$6,854,218	$6,792,967	284.13	286.15	271.56	302.76	305.53	302.80
VP SUPPORT SERVICES	$1,710,540	$8,309,400	$8,109,833	$1,832,100	$8,886,850	$9,014,952	482.82	481.51	469.95	517.13	514.98	522.40
VP FINANCE	$278,047	$1,357,604	$1,325,270	$291,548	$1,424,965	$1,472,523	68.25	68.41	66.78	71.56	71.80	74.20
VP HUMAN RESOURCES	$193,292	$956,106	$934,507	$208,604	$1,010,570	$1,038,342	49.60	49.31	49.23	53.53	53.24	54.70
SR VP/COO	$795,102	$3,833,720	$3,674,818	$855,448	$4,129,180	$4,083,131	204.03	201.96	193.59	219.51	217.53	215.10
Total Facility	$6,169,377	$30,121,490	$29,401,974	$6,737,074	$32,522,049	$32,696,816	1,493.75	1,497.01	1,460.07	1,627.98	1,612.74	1,623.60

Figure 9-4: Productivity Management—Facility Summary Report

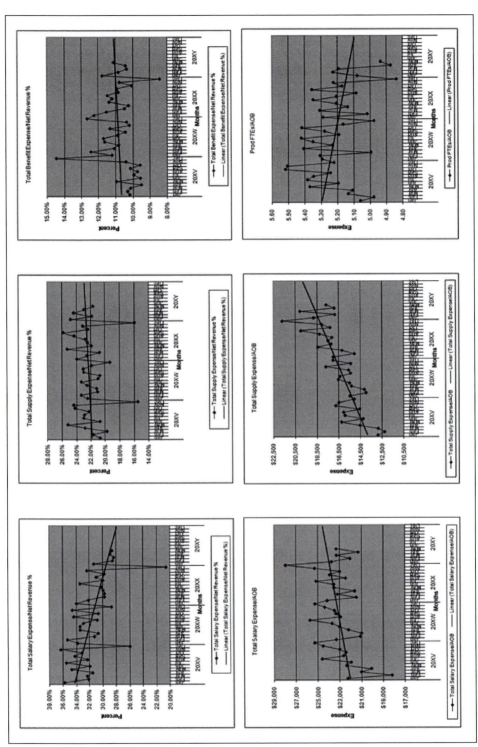

Figure 9-5: Productivity Management Scorecard Report—% Net Expense Report

- Salary expense per AOB is increasing, signaling either higher salaries or less efficient use of resources. But because overall FTEs/AOB is declining, the increase is probably caused by higher salary rate.

Many other observations can be made from these graphs. The value of reports such as this one is the ability to see indicators from different aspects of the organization, with all included on the same page, which provides a very high level overview of what is happening organization-wide. Many organizations will also include vacancy rate, turnover rates and other human resource related indicators. This allows the organization to discuss the various indicators of the organization's performance in concert with each other. Intended and sometimes unintended consequences of decisions can be seen by analyzing the different indicators together. But typically, better decision making and planning occurs when the entire business operation is understood.

Planning for the Future

The second three uses of productivity information (shown earlier in Table 9-3) are related by the ability of the department or organization to be proactive in the future. Seeing that a department is using too many resources for the workload output, the manager can use the productivity information as an impetus to identify opportunities for productivity improvement. Detailed system analysis, benchmarking, reengineering and many other process improvement tools can be applied to determine improvement opportunities. In addition, by knowing how long it takes to perform the service, expectations can be set and utilized. For example, if the typical time to complete a chest x-ray is 15 minutes, with an additional 10 minutes for the initial check-in process, a radiology department can fairly confidently tell its patients that they can expect to be in radiology for 25 minutes. Obviously, not all services can cite such definite times associated with their functions, but for those that can, such productivity information is helpful in managing patients' expectations.

Productivity information for future considerations is best used to determine future workforce needs. This need falls into two components—short-term staffing considerations and long-term work force planning. Short-term staffing issues arise when using productivity information to predict staffing needs for the near term. Short-term future staffing needs can be predicted based on projected workloads for the future (next week, next month, next six months, etc). The number of labor dollars/hours are then known, and based on a specific skill mix, can determine the number and types of positions required.

Long-term workforce planning is more interesting. By knowing the current dollars/hours per unit of measure ratios, current skill mix and projected workload volume, future staffing requirements can be estimated. Then, by applying different "what if" scenarios, such as availability or lack of a certain skill mix it minimizes, one can easily predict future workforce needs. Performing a gap analysis comparing future state with current state, a strategic plan can be developed to address the issues.

BENEFITS OF USING A PRODUCTIVITY SYSTEM

There are multiple benefits derived from using a productivity system. These include enhanced control of labor expenses, better allocation of resources, improved workforce planning, forward planning for future budgets and performance benchmarking. Each of these will be discussed next.

Control of Labor Expenses

The primary benefit of a productivity management system is that it gives organizations the ability to better manage and control labor expenses. It is imperative that these costs be controlled. The old adage, "you manage what you measure," is very appropriate here. A better understanding of the true labor expenditures of the organization is the first step in identifying areas for improvement or cost reduction. Management can identify increasing cost trends, either in a single department or throughout the entire organization, and develop an action plan to eliminate or at least slow down the increase. Implementing an action plan will lead to reduced costs, which can be tracked to the bottom line of the organization.

Allocation of Resources

A second benefit of using a productivity management system is that the system will allow for a more appropriate allocation of resources. Budget processes typically require every department in the organization to eliminate a percentage of the previous year's budget for the following year. The methodology works well, with one exception; departments that are performing well (better than budget) get penalized in comparison with their peers who are not meeting the current budget. A well-functioning productivity management system allows management to appropriately provide resources to the areas that need them and take them away from areas that do not. Also, in times of workforce shortages, management can assign resources to areas that have the most critical need first. Creative staffing assignments can be made by knowing how much labor is required to accomplish specific amounts of work at specified service levels.

Work Force Planning

A third benefit of a productivity management system is seen when critical future workforce planning activities are initiated. Changing needs within the healthcare industry, as well as the limited supply of available workers, will force organizations to begin developing their own workforces. Understanding fundamental principles surrounding productivity management will provide the basis for future workforce forecasting, including the number and skill type required. In the near future, healthcare organizations will have to invest in workforce planning efforts, and without a functioning productivity management system, will find the process very difficult, if not impossible.

Planning Future Budgets

A fourth benefit of a productivity management system is that it helps organizations prepare more realistic budgets for future years. An upward-spiraling cycle results as productivity is managed: better budgets are created; productivity is better managed, which produces even better budgets, and so on. The final result is that budgeted performance, expected performance (productivity), and actual performance converge together to produce a higher performing organization.

Benchmarking

A fifth benefit arising from the use of a productivity management system is the ability to compare an organization's performance against that of other organizations. The concept of benchmarking (discussed in more detail in Chapter 2) becomes far easier to understand and implement for organizations using productivity management systems. Once the basic concept of "you manage what you measure" is developed, the next step is to determine how well you stand up against your competitors. This leads to the concepts of process improvement and continuous process improvement. A fundamental understanding of basic productivity management concepts can help an organization become a learning organization continually striving to improve its daily operations.

NONTRADITIONAL INDICATORS

Additional Productivity Measures

As hospitals have evolved into healthcare organizations including integrated delivery systems, additional productivity measures are needed. Productivity measures are also needed for physician offices and health plans. Patient visits are the traditional physician office measure, but procedure-weighted indicators (similar to relative value units in hospital ancillary departments) are also used. Health plans need to measure multiple items, such as internal processing issues (claims processed per hour), turnaround time (time from claim to payment), rejected claims (and why), paid claims, percentage of paid and rejected claims and dollar amount of paid and rejected claims. Per member per month revenue collected and expenses paid out are vital measures of the success of health maintenance organizations. For organizations that have or will develop these functions, it is imperative that these aspects of the operations are measured and managed as well.

Software Availability

Many third-party vendor productivity systems are available for purchase. Organizations have also developed their own internal systems, using database or spreadsheet programs. These systems differ in the sophistication and level of detail they maintain, as well as their reporting capabilities (including possibilities, such as graphs, or not, multiple period reporting, or not, etc). The organization needs to understand its requirements and what it seeks from its productivity monitoring system prior to purchasing or building.

SUMMARY

Most large healthcare organizations have developed a productivity monitoring system over time. Comparing a department against itself over time and identifying significant trends is probably the most elementary application. A productivity management system uses the information that it develops in a proactive manner such as developing future budgets, improving targets and, in general, identifying areas on which to concentrate for future process improvement activities. Whether simple tools (e.g., work simplification or operations analysis) or complex tools (e.g., reengineering or benchmarking) are used, the baseline data are a product of the productivity system. Obviously staffing analyses are a direct result of applying productivity information to a specific department.

A thorough understanding of how and why productivity systems work can have a major impact on how an ME views his or her work situation. Management engineers, because of their desire to improve operations and reduce costs, typically look at the world with a belief that the "status quo can be improved" and use productivity system indicators to identify potential areas for improvement. Fundamental understanding of productivity systems leads to better understanding of staffing assignments and overall resource allocation. Knowing that increased productivity leads to reduced costs, MEs can make a significant impact on their organizations.

The concept of productivity monitoring and management is simple, yet powerful. With the ever-changing healthcare environment and the challenges that lay ahead for any healthcare organization, a refocus and emphasis on productivity management will be a requirement. A thorough understanding can help an organization and its MEs better recognize improvement opportunities. It also leads an organization to get a better handle on its labor resources. A solid understanding of productivity will lead to improved operating costs for an organization; management engineers, as productivity experts, can and should play a significant role in this change improvement.

References

1. Institute of Medicine. *To Err is Human: Building a Safer Health System.* Washington, DC: National Academy Press; 1999.
2. Gray SP, Steffy W. *Hospital Cost Containment Through Productivity Management.* New York: Van Nostrand Reinhold Co; 1983:203-208.

SECTION IV

TECHNOLOGY AND PERFORMANCE

A great deal of management and analyst time is consumed these days on issues of maximizing the value of information technology (IT). In this final part, we discuss the relationship between IT and performance and describe how engineers can contribute in these processes.

In Chapter 10, Margaret Holm, an RN and healthcare executive, describes the link between evidence-based healthcare and electronic health information systems. She discusses how the two are related today and argues for further integration in the future as healthcare evolves toward greater use of data and evidence in daily clinical decision making.

In Chapter 11, Sandra Blanke and Elizabeth McGrady, professors at the University of Dallas, describe a key process called *continuity planning,* which has as its focus the protection of resources from potential disaster. This is an area that has not received enough attention but which should become a top priority for managers and analysts. In the event of disaster, ensuring full continuity of information systems and other key processes is vital to maintaining performance during these critical times.

In Chapter 12, Guy Scalzi and Roger Kropf describe the role of service level agreements and how they can be applied in healthcare technology. This is important as management engineers frequently find themselves involved in developing and measuring service levels in projects and process improvement programs.

CHAPTER 10

Evidence-Based Healthcare and Information Systems

Margaret J. Holm

> *"Facts are stubborn things; and whatever may be our wishes, our inclinations, or the dictates of our passions, they cannot alter the state of facts and evidence."*
>
> — John Adams, former U.S. President

INTRODUCTION

A major force behind the transformation of healthcare is the use of clinical data obtained through the electronic health information system (EHIS) with the application of evidence-based healthcare (EBHC). As a result of the transformation, healthcare organizations are expected to adopt an EHIS to assist in the implementation of EBHC. The EHIS, which includes aspects such as order entry, patient records, reporting systems, access to information and decision support tools, is an important vehicle to implement required changes in healthcare delivery. **Evidence-based healthcare** incorporates the philosophy that providing quality care is based on the current *best* scientific evidence, clinical judgment and patient preference.

In an effort to reform healthcare, healthcare organizations are provided payment incentives to utilize EBHC to drive improvements in care delivery and lower healthcare cost. The payment incentives are based on clinical measures developed from the evidence and consensus by national, business and clinical leaders. As the measures are developed, healthcare organizations are putting into place an EHIS that contains EBHC tools, such as guidelines (algorithms), pathways, plans of care, medication administration records and order sets. These tools are designed to generate and capture clinical data based on EBHC and report the clinical data to the federal government and other third-party payers for reimbursement. One of the most important federal initiatives currently underway is called 'pay-for-performance,' which requires healthcare organizations and providers to obtain clinical data, which are sent electronically to third party payers. Approximately 100 private sector pay-for-performance programs are currently underway, along with several Medicare demonstration projects.[1]

Healthcare reform will occur with the assistance of the EHIS and EBHC because of the ability to quantify the value of healthcare services and exchange and compare data across organizations and individual providers. The ability to quantify the value of healthcare services has not consistently been done in the past but is now expected to transform the industry by linking the cost of a service with quality, which will eventually impact the clinical outcome. Thus, it is very important for healthcare organizations to lay a strong foundation for the development of their EHIS.

There are many variables to consider when a healthcare system is implementing an EHIS, such as software, hardware, costs, knowledge of the information technology staff, other projects within the organization that might sub-optimize the EHIS, leadership skills and governance support. However, four key variables should be considered in the planning stage to ensure that the EHIS implementation is successful and sustained:

1. The end-user's understanding of the long-term benefits and ownership of the EHIS
2. The organization's infrastructure to support implementation of the EHIS
3. National standards impacting the EHIS
4. A definition of success for each phase of implementation

END-USERS: LONG-TERM BENEFITS

The benefits of EHIS that include the use of EBHC tools are showing long-term improvements in care delivery. The Institute of Medicine (IOM) reported that with the use of information technology, medical errors could be reduced and patient safety could be improved.[2] In addition, the National Quality Forum reported studies showing benefits, through features such as the following:[1]

- Prompts that warn against the possibility of drug interaction, allergy or overdose. It also provides reminders for preventive services, such as influenza and pneumococcal vaccinations, and screening for breast, cervical, and colorectal cancer.
- Improved clinical disease tracking and compliance with clinical guidelines that lead to better outcomes.
- Accurate, up-to-date information that helps physicians keep up with new drugs as they are introduced to the market.
- Drug-specific information that eliminates confusion among drug names that sound alike.
- Improved communication between physicians and pharmacists.
- Reduced healthcare costs due to improved efficiencies.[2]

Additional studies have also demonstrated benefits. For example, Boston's Brigham and Women's Hospital showed that order entry reduced error rates by 55%, from 10.7 to 4.9 per 1000 patient-days.[3] Intermountain LDS Hospital, which is affiliated with the University of Utah Hospital in Salt Lake City, demonstrated a significant reduction in adverse drug events (ADEs) after implementation of computerized adverse drug surveillance program. The ADEs decreased from 56 ADEs to a low of 8 ADEs during a 44-month time period.[4] And, if order entry were implemented in all non-rural U.S. hospitals, it is estimated that between 570,000 and 907,000 serious medication errors could be prevented each year.[5]

With the rising costs of healthcare delivery, healthcare leaders are looking for improved ways to lower costs. According to Hillestad et al.,[6] approximately $81 billion in savings can be realized annually with large-scale implementation of the electronic health record (EHR), a component of the EHIS. And some believe that the savings could be doubled if improvements in prevention and chronic disease management were also made.[6]

Order entry is one of the most popular components of the EHIS because of the impact orders have on patient care delivery and utilization of resources. However, the upfront cost of implementing order entry is a major obstacle for many hospitals. At Brigham and Women's Hospital, the cost of developing and implementing order entry was approximately $1.9 million, with $500,000 in ongoing maintenance costs annually. Even installation of "off the shelf" order entry packages requires a significant amount of customization for each hospital and can be very expensive. It is difficult to estimate the cost of implementing order entry because of the variability in hospital size, existing level of information technology (IT) and the scope of the IT implementation project within each system. A rough estimate is in a range from $3 million to $10 million spread over several years. However, the return can be very substantial, as was the case for Brigham and Women's Hospital; the return on its initial investment has been between $5 and $10 million in annual savings.[7]

END-USERS: OWNERSHIP

Several case studies have demonstrated the significance of end-user ownership in the implementation of an EHIS. The **end-user** is the person who understands the processes, what is needed from the EHIS and the culture of the organization; therefore, it is important that he or she is involved in the initial development and supports the EHIS until it becomes a sustained activity that is integrated into the workflow. Organizations can sometimes view one aspect of the EHIS, such as order entry, as simply a software installation and determine the success of order entry by the functionality of the software product. However, it is important to note that order entry is actually creating a new process for a significant aspect of clinical care. The orders are key in defining the care to be delivered and the timing and sequence of the care to be received. It is imperative that the orders be simple and flow into or improve the existing workflow processes. Examples of how some order entry processes have been implemented follow.

In December 2005, Han et al.[8] tested their hypothesis that a commercially developed computerized practitioner order entry (CPOE) system implemented in the Children's Hospital of Pittsburgh for children requiring specialized care would reduce mortality. However, the results refuted the hypothesis by indicating an increase in mortality among the children. The authors reported that key processes were changed for patients admitted through the transport system after CPOE implementation; prior to CPOE the transport team would contact the ICU fellow and with the information from the transport team, the ICU fellow ordered critical medications for infusion. As a result, the ICU nurse would have the medications prepared prior to the patient's arrival. In addition, the ICU fellow would also order diagnostic imaging studies that the patient could receive prior to arriving in the ICU. And the full set of admission orders could be completed prior to the patient's arrival. After CPOE was implemented, the orders could not be entered into the computer system until after the patient had physically arrived, which created delays in getting the necessary treatments and tests to the patient. In addition, one physician would leave the bedside to enter the orders, leaving only one physician to attend to the unstable patient.

In 2006, Del Beccaro et al.[9] reviewed a commercially developed CPOE system within Children's Hospital and Regional Medical Center in Seattle to determine if there were any changes in risk-adjusted mortality after the implementation of CPOE in their pediatric intensive care unit. The CPOE system was implemented one year after the order entry system was implemented at Children's Hospital of Pittsburgh, and Children's Hospital (Seattle) had not found an association between CPOE and increased mortality. Prior to the "go-live," Del Beccaro then visited Children's Hospital of Pittsburgh to learn from their experience to avoid replicating the same negative workflow process changes. He concluded, "The differences in our study suggest that implementation issues (more order sets, sentences, code-set filtering, ability to get medications directly from the medication-dispensing system in emergent cases) rather than inherent issues with the CPOE itself or the underlying high risk of a particular software system are the primary risk factors affecting mortality during implementation of CPOE."[9]

In 2003, Cedar Sinai Medical Center in Los Angeles installed CPOE. After just weeks, the hospital had to withdraw CPOE because of concerns from physicians that the system was endangering patients and that it required too much work, according to the Washington Post.[10]

In 1988, the University of Virginia Medical Center in Charlottesville began implementation of a health information system. The implementation of order entry went beyond the budget and experienced delays. There were at least four issues that contributed to the organization's stress: (1) the alteration of established workflow patterns and practices; (2) literal interpretation of rules by the computer, inability of the IT system to identify intent; (3) ambiguity of governance policies; and (4) lack of a clear understanding within the physician community of the long-term strategic value of the medical information system strategy.

In 1993, Massaro[11] observed that the integration of new technology is a daily part of academic medicine; it is viewed as a natural evolutionary process. New technology is brought into the academic healthcare organization by a limited number of people who manage, understand and provide oversight of the new technology. However, for new technology such as a medical information system, it works differently in that the medical information system requires fundamental changes in the way people within the entire organization work.

All of these case examples point to the importance of integrating the end-user into the planning and development stages of the EHIS and helping him or her to understand the national agenda and the long-term benefits driving the use of the EHIS. It is also important for end-users to be a part of the change because "people issues" have proven to be more responsible for implementation failures than the technical side of the EHIS. Lewin's "field theory"[12] suggests that to motivate people, they need to be involved in making the change. When they are not involved, they will resist because of concern that the change might be negative. As Lorenzi et al.[13] state, "If the group members perceive that they own the problem and the solution, they will work with the developers to make the system work."

NATIONAL STANDARDS

The healthcare industry is rapidly moving to capture essential data related to the primary business of healthcare, which is clinical care delivery and patient outcomes. To move this effort more quickly, the federal government is requiring the development of the EHR. In April 2004, President George W. Bush called for widespread use of health information technology and for EHRs to be in use for most Americans by year 2014. In addition, Secretary of the Department of Health and Human Services (HHS) Mike Leavitt announced, "Information is a pivotal part of transforming our healthcare system. Working in close collaboration, the federal government and private sector can drive changes that will lead to fewer medical errors, lower costs, less hassle and better care."[14]

Because of the significance of EHR implementation, the government has provided funding and developed an infrastructure to ensure that this initiative moves forward. Since May 2005, there have been more than twelve bills introduced pertaining to the EHR with focus on development and adoption. In addition, there was a $61.7 million appropriation for HHS designated specifically to address the nationwide infrastructure.[14] Further, the National Institute of Health launched an initiative to create an informatics infrastructure for collaboration with cancer and biomedical research communities. This initiative will provide open-source software and information to enable research to move to the bedside at a more rapid pace.[15]

The Office of the National Coordinator for Health Information Technology (ONC) and the American Health Information Community (AHIC) were established in 2004 by HHS with the goal of improving healthcare through IT. The focus and goal of ONC is to develop a certification process for health information technology products developed by the private sector. Thus, the Certification Commission for Healthcare Information Technology (CCHIT) was created. The mission of CCHIT is to accelerate the adoption of health information technology by creating an efficient, credible and sustainable product certification program. The goals of CCHIT product certification are to:

- Reduce the risk of healthcare IT investment by physicians and other providers.
- Ensure interoperability (compatibility) of healthcare IT products.
- Assure payers and purchasers providing incentives for electronic health record adoption that the return on investment (ROI) will be improved quality.
- Protect the privacy of patients' personal health information.

The standards created from the CCHIT focus on functionality, interoperability, security and reliability for the ambulatory and inpatient settings. The standards are specific and detailed, with some of the key elements of the criteria described next.[16]

Functionality

Functionality is defined by CCHIT as setting features and functions to meet a basic set of requirements. Some of the requirements include patient problem list, allergy and adverse reactions list, patient history, consents and authorizations, supporting standard care plans, guidelines, protocols, order sets, notifications and reminders for disease management, prevention services and wellness, ordering medications, supporting notifications for drug interactions, ordering diagnostic tests, managing results, providing rules-driven financial and administrative coding assistance.

Interoperability

Interoperability is defined by CCHIT as enabling standards-based data exchange with other sources of healthcare information. Sharing information via a common electronic language with other organizations or databases for the accumulation of multiple data from multiple sites will allow for a view of geographic areas, larger sample sizes and other uses from common databases. As the federal government moves interoperability to the forefront for the EHIS, there is the potential for workflow within healthcare organizations to change due to the influence of data on the operations of healthcare delivery. With data coming across the continuum of care, each sector of care delivery will be impacted: ambulatory, emergency, acute and post-acute services.

Security and Reliability

Security requires data privacy and robustness to prevent data loss. The importance of data security is becoming clearer as individuals can be inconvenienced or harmed when data are not used as intended.

Reliability ensures that the system works consistently every time and without experiencing delays or interruptions in service.

National healthcare standards are being set by the Leapfrog Group, which comprises representatives from large corporations throughout the country. One of the first safety standards chosen by the Leapfrog Group is practitioner order entry; the standard states "orders are integrated with patient information, including laboratory and prescription data. The order is then automatically checked for potential errors or problems."

In order to fully meet Leapfrog's standard, hospitals must meet the following criteria:

1. Ensure that physicians enter at least 75% of medication orders via a computer system that includes prescribing-error prevention software.
2. Demonstrate that their inpatient order entry system can alert physicians of at least 50% of common, serious prescribing errors, using a testing protocol now under development by First Consulting Group and the Institute for Safe Medication Practices.
3. Require that physicians electronically document a reason for overriding an interception prior to doing so.

The Leapfrog Group has developed a survey, available on their Web site, for healthcare organizations to determine the current level of IT activity within their organizations. The survey assists healthcare organizations in planning their EHIS.

Another important organization setting standards for the EHIS is the National Quality Forum, which has identified electronic health information as critical to providing care that is safe, effective and delivered in an efficient manner. The EHIS provides clinicians with complete patient information and facilitates compliance with evidence-based practice guidelines, better coordination and management of patients with chronic conditions, optimized medication prescribing and administration, reduced redundancy of laboratory and imaging services with increased accuracy in coding and more timely billing for services.[1]

It is important for the end-user to know of the changes the federal government is putting into place in order to better understand the long-term benefits of the EHIS. Examples of these changes include: monitoring medication administration, notifications of patient information, and decision-making tools. The end-user will receive information about individual patients and groups of patients. The information can assist them in making changes to improve care and for easier implementation of EBHC.

INFORMATION TECHNOLOGY INFRASTRUCTURE

The solidity of the infrastructure within an organization that develops and coordinates the work associated with IT is key to long-term sustainability of efforts to implement an EHIS. A key leader for this work typically is the chief information officer (CIO), who reports directly to the chief executive officer. Committees comprising representatives from various areas, including clinicians are established to prioritize the capital expenditures, software installations and other resource expenditures. They also formulate a plan to integrate this new technology into the workflow.

Plans for IT development within a healthcare organization have been found to be similar around the country. In 2006, HIMSS Analytics, a research subsidiary of the Healthcare Information and Management Systems Society, identified healthcare organizations at various stages of development for an EHR, a component of the EHIS (see Figure 10-1). Fifty percent of the healthcare organizations had developed a clinical data repository in which the ancillary clinical systems feed into one large data repository. Twenty-one percent had laboratory, pharmacy, radiology and ancillary clinical systems that stand-alone and do not feed into a clinical data repository.

An emerging IT infrastructure for healthcare is the service-oriented architecture (SOA), currently seen in the finance industry and now moving to healthcare. With SOA, the design is made to link computational resources based on the customer's needs, allowing many diverse servers under different ownership. The purpose is to offer uniform methods for servers to interact with one another in a consistent, dependable environment. SOA is in a stage of evolution, in the same way as Web services architecture continues to evolve, which is by connecting with more information faster and with more reliability. For healthcare organizations that have independent clinical databases within departments, the SOA will allow for cross-utilization of the data.

One of the most important aspects of the EHIS is that it allows the clinician the ability to obtain information to aid in decision making. For clinicians, clinical performance is tied to the ability to obtain information from the patient, objectively and subjectively, and to assess, diagnosis and name the most accurate, up-to-date interventions. All of this is to occur at a specific point in time in order for care to be delivered in an effective and efficient manner. At the same time, clinicians must be able to document their findings, plans of care, and orders for others to follow in helping to treat the patient.

It is from these actions that care is provided to the patient and clinical information about the patient is obtained. These actions often occur in a hurried situation inside a busy hospital or clinic where there is little time for the clinician to reflect or think about

Stage	Key Events	% Adoption
Stage 7	Hospital has paperless EMR environment; Capable of sharing data with a regional network	0%
Stage 6	Full physician documentation and charting; full clinical decision support; full PACS	<1%
Stage 5	Closed-loop medication administration	<1%
Stage 4	CPOE available for use by any practitioner; clinical protocols	2%
Stage 3	Clinical documentation; first-level clinical decision support; PACS available outside Radiology	8%
Stage 2	Ancillary Clinical Systems feed to a clinical data repository	50%
Stage 1	Laboratory, Pharmacy, Radiology, Ancillary Clinical Systems exist	21%
Stage 0	Some clinical automation, but all three ancillary clinical systems not installed	19%

Source: HIMSS Analytics, 2006; National Quality Forum, 2007.

Figure 10-1: Hospital Stages of EHR Adoption

what to order. EBHC tools give clinicians the ability to visually identify the treatments indicated for a particular disease, symptom or research protocol.

As we learn more about how clinicians think and the ever-increasing volumes of information which they are required to know, it is apparent that EBHC tools will become more significant. Such tools will continue to evolve over time to further support clinical decision making by collecting data for process and outcome analysis.

Various tools in different formats are available: guidelines, algorithms, info-buttons, pathways, e-prescribing and order sets. Guidelines and algorithms provide the clinician with information on how to best treat the disease or symptom based on the evidence or consensus of experts in a related field. Info-buttons provide quick answers on specific clinical topics in a concise format to help the clinician rapidly obtain information. Pathways describe key interventions found in the guidelines in more detail and in a sequential fashion to drive outcomes and give caregivers and patients a road map of what to expect over time. The medication prescriptions are entered and electronically transmitted to the pharmacy. The order sets are unique, for they drive the actions related to the care that will be delivered by the healthcare team. Order sets can impact patient safety, workflow processes, and reimbursement.

With order sets the clinician can perform the following functions:

- View a template that contains key evidence-based or research protocol components of treatments or tests that pertain to that particular disease or symptom. The clinician decides if these elements are right for his or her patient at a particular point in time. The order set provides the clinician with visual cues rather than having to think of all of the treatments or tests from memory.
- Engage in a consistent method of communication among the healthcare delivery team to reduce medical errors and increase patient safety.
- Pause when an alert is given in order to take time to rethink before ordering.
- Increase the speed of the ordering process by electronically notifying the lab, radiology, nutrition services and pharmacy of his or her order.

As we move to rapidly capture clinical data, we rely on the bedside caregivers to provide their observations and readings as part of their workflow. There are organizations that are moving forward to further develop this technology. At Columbia University in New York City, Dr. Bakken is exploring the use of nursing order entry through the handheld tool, called i-APN, which is carried in the clinician's pocket. The handheld tool contains the order set and allows for order entry in a simple fashion by focusing on only five areas: diagnosis, procedure, treatment, patient teaching and patient referral.[18]

As part of an organization's infrastructure for IT, there should be mechanisms to manage the introduction of new technologies with concurrent changes in workflow and culture. Senior management plays a valuable role in this effort and is expected to be able to describe the new vision of patient care and how patient EHIS will be a part of that new vision. In addition, senior leaders will be called on to sustain the course, through supporting the organization's culture, developing the champions, finding the resources, removing the barriers and promoting the milestones of the work achieved thus far. It is a multi-year commitment and sometimes takes years before clinical improvements are noted; therefore, the sustainability of the plan primarily rests with senior leaders.

DEFINING SUCCESS

Evaluation of the EHIS is often overlooked, or it is evaluated independently as a technical system, not as a structural change integrated into the workflow to achieve the desired benefit. Therefore, it is important to complete an evaluation that reviews all of the components of the implementation of the EHIS: workflow design, end-user satisfaction, risks, costs and the technical review.

With any change, the underlying motive is the belief that the change will provide benefit. The definition of benefit for a particular EHIS project will create the actions driving the project. The decision of how to define the benefit resides with the people creating the plan for change. Examples of benefit include improving patient outcomes, easing the workload, answering questions, reducing risks, gaining data for decision making, and lowering costs.

After the intended benefit is defined, the focus will need to be on the measures that will be used to evaluate the benefit. The design of the measures can be either quantitative or qualitative, or both. Identifying the origin of the data that comprise the measures and any assumptions associated with the data will yield better information for decision making. With each phase of implementation, the organizational leaders should define the measure of success for the EHIS and then evaluate for each. This will give the leaders an opportunity to redesign workflow processes to apply to the next phase of implementation.[19]

SUMMARY

The expectations for healthcare leaders to improve care and lower costs were in place before the prospective payment system emerged for acute care in 1983. The expectations continue to this day; however, in the current environment, clinical data will be the driving force that will improve care and lower costs. The clinical data will be derived from an EHIS incorporating the evidence. Making these changes requires forethought and implementing mechanisms of sustainability. Therefore, it is important for healthcare leaders to understand these key factors when implementing an EHIS: (1) the end-user's understanding of the long-term benefits and ownership of the EHIS; (2) the organization's infrastructure to support implementation of EHIS; (3) national standards impacting the EHIS; and (4) a definition of success for each phase of implementation.

References

1. National Quality Forum. CEO Survival Guide to Electronic Health Record Systems. July 4, 2007. Available at www.nqfexecutiveinstitute.org.

2. Institute of Medicine; Dick RS, Steen EB (eds). *The Computer-Based Patient Record: An Essential Technology for Healthcare.* Washington, DC: National Academy Press; 1991.

3. Bates DW, Lucian L, Cullen D, et al. Effect of computerized physician entry and a team intervention on prevention of serious medication errors. *JAMA.* 1998; 280: 811-1816.

4. Evans RS, Pestotnik SL, Classen DC, et al. Preventing adverse drug events in hospitalized patients. *Annals of Pharmacotherapy.* 1994 (April 28); 4:523-527.

5. Poon EG, Blumenthal D, Jaggi T, et al. Overcoming barriers to adopting and implementing computerized physician order entry systems in U.S. hospitals. *Health Affairs.* 2004; 23:184-190.

6. Hillestad R, Bigelow J, Bower A, et al. Can electronic medical record systems transform healthcare? Potential health benefits, savings, and costs. *Health Affairs.* 2005; 4:1103-1117.

7. Birkmeyer CM, Lee J, Bates DW, et al. Will electronic order entry reduce healthcare costs? *Effective Clinical Practice.* 2002; 5:67-74.

8. Han YY, Carcillo JA, Venkataraman ST, et al. Unexpected increased mortality after implementation of a commercially sold computerized physician order entry system. *Pediatrics.* 2005; 116(6):1506-1512.

9. Del Beccaro MA, Jeffries HE, Eisenberg MA, Harry ED. Computerized provider order entry implementation: No association with increased mortality rates in an intensive care unit. *Pediatrics.* 2006; 118:290-295.

10. Connolly C. Cedars-Sinai doctors cling to pen and paper. *Washington Post.* March 21, 2005. at www.gunston.doit.gmu.edu/healthscience/740/Presentations/cedars-sinai%20cpoe%20washpost%203-21-05.pdf. Accessed online on February 10, 2008.

11. Massaaro TA. Introducing physician order entry at a major academic medical center. *Academic Medicine.* 1993; 68:20-30.

12. Lewin K. *Field Theory in Social Science: Selected Theoretical Papers.* D. Cartwright. New York: Harper & Row; 1951.

13. Lorenzi NM, Riley RT, et al. Antecedents of the people and organizational aspects of medical informatics: Review of the literature. *Journal of American Medical Informatics Association.* 1997; (April) 4:79-92.

14. Health and Human Services, Leavitt M. HHS Secretary and Leading U.S. Companies Say Health Information Technology Should be Urgent Priority (press release). May 11, 2005. Available at www.hhs.gov/news/press/2005press/20050511.html.

15. National Cancer Institute. Cancer Biomedical Informatics Grid. Available at www.cabig.nci.nih.gov. Accessed July 4, 2007.

16. Certification Commission for Healthcare Information Technology. Certification for HIT vendors. May 29, 2007. Available at www.cchit.org/about/.

17. The LeapFrog Group. Computerized Physician Order Entry. Available at www.leapfroggroup.org. Accessed July 4, 2007.

18. Bakken S. National Library of Medicine, Bioinformatics Course. Spring, 2007. Woodshole, MA.

19. Ash JS, Sittig DF, Poon EG, et al. The extent and importance of unintended consequences related to computerized provider order entry. *Journal of American Medical Informatics Association.* 2007; 4:415-23.

CHAPTER 11

A Performance-Based Approach to Continuity Planning

Sandra Blanke and Elizabeth McGrady

> *"Continuity does not rule out fresh approaches to fresh situations."*
> — Dean Rusk, former U.S. Secretary of State

INTRODUCTION

Hospitals serve as sentinels of refuge in times of disaster, as demonstrated by the influx of residents to hospitals during Hurricane Katrina. Therefore, it is imperative that hospitals and other healthcare organizations and providers remain operable during all conditions. With only 24% of general hospitals actually owned by state or local governments,[1] it is difficult to establish and enforce standards or mandate and control interoperability of healthcare resources in response to disaster.

There is also minimal connectivity between the public health system and healthcare providers. Though nearly $8 billion has been allocated to disaster preparedness by the U.S. Congress since 2002, a study conducted by PricewaterhouseCoopers' Health Research Institute[2] found disaster response planning by the healthcare system to be fragmented and disjointed. The study also reported that fewer than 20% of primary care physicians stated they were well prepared to respond to a disaster.

The priority focus of all healthcare providers is taking care of patients. This unified focus of purpose may also contribute to managers' resistance to diverting attention and resources to longer term organizational needs, such as continuity planning and disaster recovery. Yet these management functions can help ensure sustainability and mitigate interruption of services.[3] Healthcare continuity plans should address command, communications, patient triage, and flow and security as part of their emergency preparedness effort. Continuity planning is necessary for all healthcare organizations, whether large multi-facility systems or small agencies or single provider practices.

DISASTER REDEFINED

Disasters come in many forms and sizes. A disaster may be a catastrophic fire or a hurricane that renders a building or even an entire city inoperable. Alternatively, a disaster may be as simple as the loss of power to one building or one part of a building due to a single tree falling. The point is, although it is certain that other disasters will occur, there is no certainty as to the time, place, form or size of the events. Adequate continuity and disaster response planning are critical to ensure that healthcare organizations are able to serve patients even during adverse situations.

We will define key terms first in order to establish meaning before discussing these issues. According to Wells et al.,[4] a **disaster** is defined as "any occurrence that can have a detrimental effect on an organization either in whole or in part" that disrupts the organization's ability to function. Examples of disasters include accidents, failed technology and acts of nature.

Disaster recovery is defined as "minimizing the effects of a disaster and taking the necessary steps to ensure that the resources, personnel and business processes are able to resume operation in a timely manner."[5] Disaster recovery includes providing methods and procedures for dealing with the disaster and its immediate aftermath.

Continuity planning is "providing methods and procedures for dealing with longer-term outages and disasters."[5] Continuity planning includes performing business in a different mode and dealing with customers, partners and shareholders through different channels until regular conditions are back in place.

Healthcare continuity planning has evolved as systems have had to cope with what are often unpredictable and sometimes large-scale events. Coastal hospitals learned many lessons from the devastation wrought by Hurricanes Hugo (Charleston, South Carolina, 1989) and Andrew (Miami, Florida, 1992), but the unprecedented level of flooding that occurred as a result of Hurricane Katrina brought new lessons in disaster response, not only at the disaster site but also in remote locales, as masses of people were transferred to other cities such as Dallas and Houston. Healthcare providers in these cities had to respond to immediate medical needs, such as medication resupply for patients without medical records and whose medical practitioners were also relocated elsewhere and not able to be contacted.

The Oklahoma City bombing of a government building (1995) and the September 11, 2001 terrorist attacks on the World Trade Center in New York City forced the need for increased healthcare surge capacity from non-weather related events. Following the Oklahoma City event, St. Anthony's Hospital in Oklahoma City treated 500 victims injured in the bombing, and, following the World Trade Center attack, Saint Vincent's Catholic Medical Center in New York City treated more than 800 patients.[6] The US Department of Health and Human Services (HHS) defines **surge capacity** as "the ability to rapidly expand beyond normal services to meet increased demand for qualified personnel, medical care and public health in the event of bioterrorism or other large-scale public health emergencies or disasters."[6]

Despite lessons learned from past disasters and the inadequacies of current readiness, a revisiting of an ancient phenomenon—pandemic infection—may produce the biggest challenge to date. In the event of mass infection, the provision of healthcare services will indeed become local, as the federal government will not be able to simultaneously respond to multiple sites. In the Department of Homeland Security 2006 report,[7] the U.S. government outlined six responsibilities of the government in response to a potential bird flu epidemic:

1. Containment
2. Guidance regarding protective measures
3. Modifications to laws and regulations to facilitate response
4. Modification of monetary policy
5. Procurement and distribution of vaccines and antiviral medications
6. Research and development of vaccines and medications

It will be up to individual communities to take care of their citizens. This new version of an old disaster is forecasted to occur in two waves that may span a period of 18 months. A gap of between 9 and 12 months exists between the time that the human-to-human strain of the flu is identified and the time the vaccine can be produced and distributed to mass populations.[9] With 30% of the population sick and healthcare employee absenteeism estimated at between 20% and 30% during this period, individual hospitals will not be unable to respond to the magnitude of the disaster and, therefore, must plan accordingly.

However, despite the dramatic response required by a major catastrophe and given the trend of outside funding focused on bioterrorism, it is more likely that a healthcare organization will face a more commonplace event, such as fire or loss of electrical power. The Visiting Nurses Association (VNA) of North Texas experienced a devastating fire to their multi-story facility. Brit Carpenter, president and CEO, immediately focused on the survival and evacuation of those in the building with a second focus on continuing care and services while working through the elements of the disaster. The VNA had a disaster recovery plan and was immediately able to continue operations. Key elements to the success of the VNA included a strategy to address each of the following questions:

1. What is the immediate impact that will occur?
2. How will we communicate when the normal communications method is not available?
3. Where are important telephone numbers stored, and what is the back-up location?
4. Who is responsible for work scheduling during the disaster? How will employees get their work schedules?
5. Where are back-up supplies, or how can they be purchased during the disaster?
6. What is the back-up process for all data and services, including billing, payroll, payments to vendors, patient records, statutory reporting, etc?
7. Where are important insurance documents stored? Are all items properly insured and listed? What the deductibles? Who is the carrier? (This would include any other important insurance questions.)
8. How can working capital be accessed, and how will the financial part of the business continue to operate during and following the disaster? (For all not-for-profits it is important that donors know their funding is critical at this time.) Is there a back-up process for collections and tracking of contributions during times of disaster?
9. Did the disaster occur as a result of any negligence or fault, and is there a need to contact any legal agency?

The continuity plan should address these key issues for the most likely or most critical events.

STRATEGIC APPROACH

Disaster planning begins as a strategic imperative, with strategy that involves the allocation and deployment of organizational resources. The governance of the organization must decide on the allocation of resources for disaster planning, mitigation and response. In an era of scarce capital and cash resources, mandates to provide care for the uninsured, and the need to maintain a technological advantage and competitive "service-scape," it is tempting to ignore resource allocation in continuity planning.

Once an assessment and plan are complete, investments to improve disaster response, such as changes in facility or physical plant infrastructure, may be cost prohibitive. For example, during Hurricane Hugo (1989), although hospitals discovered the risk of placing fuel storage tanks below ground and power generators and electrical conduits at ground level and subsequently shared this knowledge, hospitals in New Orleans suffered the same problems during Hurricane Katrina.[10]

Even when solutions to mitigate identified problems are known, their implementation may be cost prohibitive. For example, a pilot project on constructing flexible facilities to accommodate volume surges estimated an additional construction cost of 30%, a considerable obstacle.[11] In some cases, federal funding is available to offset cost. While certain hospitals have received an estimated $80,000 each from the agency Health Resources and Services Administration after 2001, it is far less than the necessary outlay.[12]

Governing bodies must decide how continuity planning recommendations fit within overall strategic direction. As part of its mission as a major referral center, the University of Nebraska Medical Center made a strategic decision to spend $1 million, three quarters of which was financed by federal funds, for a 10-bed unit to respond to infectious disease outbreak. Associated operating costs for training and staffing at the new facility represented $165,000 per year.[8] The magnitude of the need is so great and diverse that it is not possible to plan for all contingencies, and therefore healthcare organizations must prioritize their focus and resource allocation.

Once strategic direction is provided, the organization can proceed with the following analysis conducted on three levels. First, those with responsibility for specific areas should follow the seven-step model for their areas. Second, administration should assign responsibility to an individual or team for assembling the departmental continuity plans into a master document and planning for the organization as a whole. Third, the organizational plan should include full interoperability with the community it serves.

HOW READY IS READY?

The Joint Commission (previously called the Joint Commission on Accreditation of Healthcare Organizations or JCAHO) publishes standards for compliance with emergency preparedness. Their standards require development of a written emergency operations plan that includes mitigation of hazards, preparedness, response and recovery. The standards require integration of organizational plans with overall community initiatives and annual review. They recommend that organizations develop plans to either stockpile or have access to supplies sufficient to operate for 96 hours and to contract with an alternative site for care. Selection of this site requires careful consideration regarding the type of emergency most likely to occur. For example, a hospital in New Orleans had a contract to transfer patients to Hattiesburg, Mississippi, as part of its hurricane preparedness but Katrina was such a mammoth and powerful storm that even hospitals that far inland were preparing for disaster as well and could not receive the transfers. Organizations must consider the type and magnitude of potential disasters in selecting repair and service contracts.

Although these are helpful minimum standards for hospitals, many healthcare organizations do not participate in The Joint Commission accreditation process; therefore, use of the following tools by any healthcare organization will be helpful in such situations and are designed to address basic problems, yet are comprehensive enough to benefit all types and sizes of organizations.

In a recent study, 96% of managers of non-profit organizations, including healthcare organizations surveyed, acknowledged the need for continuity planning and disaster recovery training.[13] Continuity planning was deemed to be a critical success factor in supporting clients in times of disaster, with the top continuity planning need being overall training. The open-ended responses for training and preparation needs with response frequency are listed in Table 11-1.

Table 11-1: List of Training Preparation Needs

Training Preparation Needs	Percent
Overall planning training	50.0
Communication during disaster	14.6
Development of plans	10.4
Ability to coordinate and link with other organizations	10.4
Ability to find resources	6.3
Internal prioritization and coordination	6.3
Evacuation/relocation	2.0

The University of Dallas Information Assurance program and Nonprofit Leadership Institute used the survey results to develop a Seven-Step Continuity Planning (CP) training tool.[13] The tool was tested with Dallas (Texas)-area organizations. The CP training tool includes the following steps in sequential order:

1. Assess the readiness level of the organization
2. Determine likely risk
3. Conduct an impact analysis (IA)
4. Develop an emergency response
5. Create an organizational resumption plan
6. Test and audit the plan
7. Perform plan maintenance

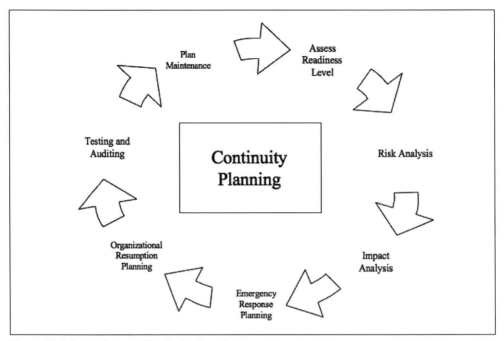

Figure 11-1: Seven Steps to Continuity Planning

Continuity planning is an ongoing process and requires reassessment at least annually or when significant changes occur in the organization. Such planning includes the following:

- Taking a longer look at the problem
- Getting the right people to the right places
- Offering service in a different mode until normal conditions are back in place
- Responding to clients, volunteers, board members, vendors and others through different channels until normality returns

Figure 11-1 and the sections that follow are provided to depict the actual steps in a circular and continuous flow.

STEP 1: ASSESS READINESS LEVEL

In a 2007 study, 60% of community not-for-profit organizations reported they had a continuity and disaster recovery plan in place and 40% did not.[13] Of organizations that had a plan, only 13% had reviewed, updated and tested the plan in the last year. There is a critical difference in having a plan and thoroughly implementing the planning process.

The recommended first step of the plan is for organizations to assess their preparedness (readiness) for a disaster. This can be accomplished by measuring their Readiness Index score based on the 14-item list below. The score is measured by affirmative response for completion of each of the following items:

- Having a disaster recovery plan in place
- Identification of threats
- Identification of probabilities of threats
- Identification of vulnerabilities

- Identification of potential impact of vulnerabilities
- Annual review of plan
- Annual update of plan
- Annual testing of plan
- Key contact list
- Electronic storage of plan
- Location of plan known by multiple staff
- Location of alternate location for conducting services
- Executing repair and service contracts
- Communication of plan with reciprocal organizations

The mean score for the Readiness Index in the 2007 study was 6.2 of a possible score of 14.0, indicating that although organizations have initiated the continuity and disaster planning process, there is still work to be done for most organizations.[14] Healthcare organizations participating in the study exceeded the average with a score of 9.7 but still fell short of the target score of 14.0. Organizations can use the Readiness Index as a means of charting and communicating progress within the organization and as a means to tracking progress of community partners. Communities can use the Readiness Index to track the overall preparedness level and to identify areas of vulnerability and additional training needed.

STEP 2: PERFORM RISK ANALYSIS

The next step is to complete a risk analysis. **Risk** is defined as the possibility of a person or entity suffering harm or loss.[4] **Risk analysis** is the process of analyzing threats and vulnerabilities.[13] There are four strategies for managing or mitigating risk based on the risk priority. The strategies are avoidance, correction, transference and acceptance. Avoidance is accomplished by eliminating or entirely avoiding the risk. The best way to avoid an Internet computer virus risk is to not access the Internet. Although this is generally not possible or realistic, the next most reasonable approach is to implement a correction. The correction may be to maintain current anti-virus software, utilize personal firewalls and implement a policy to not open e-mails and attachments from individuals that are not known to the recipient.

Transference is accomplished by transferring the risk to a third party. Car, home and flood insurance policies are purchased for the purpose of transferring risk to the insurance company. Acceptance of the risk is a strategy in which the cost of the risk is considered and compared with the benefit of the solution. If accepting the risk is less risky or less costly than the necessary solution, then accepting the risk may a reasonable decision. An example of risk acceptance is when an organization decides to self-insure and does not purchase third-party insurance.

With these four risk strategies for mitigating and managing risk in mind, the organization will begin the risk analysis phase. In this phase each functional area and the organization as a whole will describe and prioritize all services performed (Table 11-2), prepare an inventory of assets (Table 11-3), prioritize disasters and threats based on historical information (Table 11-4), estimate the likelihood of the threat occurrence (Table 11-5) and assess the impact to the organization if the disaster occurs (Table 11-6).

Each item will be prioritized by assigning a level of importance using a scale of one to ten, with ten signifying the greatest importance and one the least importance. While the priority contribution is a subjective scale, assigning relative significance can differentiate the importance of items. Participants must be cautioned from assigning high scores to each item. The following tables are examples for the information system functional area.

Table 11-2: Services Performed

Service	Description	Priority Contribution Scale (10=most important)
Patient registration system	Patient information	10
Medical records	Patient medical information	9
Decision system support	Organizational metrics	5
Supply chain system	Supply vendors, orders	8
Human resources systems	Staff/position information	9
Volunteer information	Volunteer records	5

Assets

Assets are items of value to the organization and may include highly trained healthcare workers. Because healthcare organizations may serve as first responders, their assets may be placed in harm's way. Assets may be jeopardized by the response to disaster in addition to the disaster itself. New York-Presbyterian Hospital lost four employees, seven ambulances and two service delivery vehicles in response to the emergency at the World Trade Center on September 11, 2001.[12] In addition to inventorying existing assets, organizations should determine the need for additional assets such as decontamination or bio-containment facilities. Assets may be grouped into categories for simplification. Table 11-3 provides a sample format and content information for clarification of possible assets.

Table 11-3: Asset Inventory

Asset Inventory	Description	Priority Contribution—Criticality (scale of 1–10)
Computer hardware	Mainframe, servers, PCs	8
Computer patient software	Patient data	8
Computer word processing	Word processing	4
Computer – facility	Locations of hardware	8
Generator	Emergency power source	10
IS employees	Technicians	10

These functional areas should then be incorporated into a master plan. The master plan may reprioritize areas of criticality based on overall need.

Threats

The next step in risk analysis is to identify likely threats based on historical information and anticipated future occurrences. A **threat** is described as an impending danger or harm that can result in an undesired event. Threats are grouped into four categories including human, forces of nature, infrastructure and technology.

In using these categories to complete this section of the continuity plan, individuals and teams will be able to focus planning toward the most likely specific threat occurrences. While the September 11 attack, the East Coast power outage, the 2005 Hurricanes Rita and Katrina may come to mind first, it is important to remember that natural disasters represent approximately only one percent of all serious interruptions.[14] Though their impact may be the greatest, their likelihood is lowest. The threat of a loss of electricity is more likely a real threat and one that should be on the threat list of every organization. Table 11-4 provides a framework and sample content information for clarification of possible threats.

Table 11-4: Threat Identification (Sample)

Threat Source	Threat	Asset	Service/Group Affected
Force of nature (tree fell on power line during strong winds)	Loss of electricity	Hardware	All information systems not powered by generator
Human	Important files deleted on the computer system	Software	Medical records
Human (spark from welder caused fire in building)	Fire	Hardware	All information systems
Infrastructure outdated	Flood (broken pipe)	Computing facility	All information systems
Human—deliberate	Physical vandalism or sabotage	Hardware, software, data	All information systems

Once services, assets and threats are identified, the actual analysis can begin. The items in Tables 11-2 through 11-4 are used to import data into a threat-to-asset likelihood analysis (Table 11-5) and a threat-to-asset impact analysis review (Table 11-6). The organization will use the threats and assets identified in Table 11-3 and the information in Table 11-4 in conjunction with the experience and knowledge of the staff to assign the likelihood of occurrence. The purpose of this table is to provide a master table that identifies the threats, assets and the likelihood of occurrence. The sample information is provided in Table 11-5.

The impact of the threat to the asset is utilized to determine the severity of the threat. Again, the expertise of the organization is used to assess and log assets and impact in Table 11-6.

Table 11-5: Threats-to-Asset Likelihood

Threat	Asset	Likelihood of Occurrence (1–10, 10=most likely)
Loss of electricity	Perishable foods and drugs	8
Important files deleted on the computer system	Computer data and medical records	7
Fire	Mainframe and PCs	5
Flood (broken pipe)	Computing facility	4
Physical vandalism or sabotage	Software	3
Bird flu	IS technicians	3

Table 11-6: Threats-to-Asset Impact

Threat	Asset	Impact
Loss of electricity	Perishable foods and drugs	10
Important files deleted on the computer system	Computer data	8
Fire	Kitchen appliances (e.g., refrigerators, freezers)	10
Flood (broken pipe)	Computing facility	10
Physical vandalism	Software	4
Bird flu	IS technicians	10

STEP 3: IMPACT ANALYSIS – RISK PRIORITIZATION

The impact analysis (IA) determines the impact of threats to the organization's assets and services. The IA table is built utilizing information from the multiple tables created in the risk analysis phase. In step 3, the IA objective is to prioritize how risk to the asset or service impacts the individual departments within the organization. For example, a threat that keeps the accounting department from being able to process payroll or pay vendor accounts payable will most likely be deemed a higher risk than a threat that keeps the staff from being able to print contracts for a short period of time.

Table 11-7 utilizes examples of threats and assets as were utilized in prior tables. Then Criticality is utilized from Table 11-3, Likelihood from Table 11-5 and Impact from Table 11-6. The risk priority formula in Table 11-7 is calculated as follows:

$$\text{Risk Priority} = \text{Criticality} + \text{Likelihood} + \text{Impact}$$

Risk priority is an important value in that it provides the organization with a numeric value that has been methodically derived through the various tables in step 2. The risk priority indicates the area of resource focus and prioritization to be utilized when preparing for the most critical, likely disaster situations with the greatest potential impact.

Table 11-7: Business Impact Analysis – Risk Prioritization

Threat	Asset/Service	Criticality	Likelihood	Impact	Risk Priority
Loss of electricity	Perishable food and drugs	10	8	10	25
Deletion of files	Computers	8	7	8	23
Fire	Mainframe and PCs	8	5	10	23
Flood (broken pipe)	Computing facility	5	4	10	19
Physical Vandalism	Software	5	3	4	12
Bird flu	Employees	10	3	10	23

STEP 4: EMERGENCY RESPONSE PLANNING

The emergency response plan (ERP) documents preparation for events that threaten the safety and security of the organization's assets, operational functions and resources. The ERP defines the action steps to be taken while the emergency or disaster is in progress. The most important questions for an ERP plan are: What do I do now; who do I contact; what do I document and on what forms?

Independent of the type or size of the organization it is critical to have an emergency response team (ERT) or an emergency response individual (ERI) in the case of smaller operations. The ERT will include staff members, department heads and front-line individual contributors who are intimately familiar with the responsibilities of the organization. The function of the ERP team is to create the ERP plan, test and maintain the plan and enact the plan in the event of an emergency.

In order to determine who should be on the ERT, the tables in step 2 can be utilized as a reminder of expertise utilized to perform the services, the individuals most familiar with the assets and possibly individuals that have had prior emergency or disaster training. A sample of the team list is provided in Table 11-8.

Table 11-8: Emergency Contact Listing

Name	Department	Responsibilities	Contact Information
John Doe	Payroll	Collect time sheets and create bi-weekly payroll	Telephone number, e-mail and address
Mary Smith	Food Services	Prepare food for the patients and staff	Telephone number, e-mail and address
Henry Retz	Building Services	Contact to building utilities companies, electrical shut off, building water systems	Telephone number, e-mail and address
Betsy Jones	Public Affairs	Communicate with the news media	Telephone number, e-mail and address
Elizabeth Grace	Information Management	Computers, computer systems, phone lines, back-up copies of data, remote data copies, others	Telephone number, e-mail and address

Effective communication is a key issue in disaster response. Lessons learned by healthcare teams who responded to the September 11 attack dictate the need for redundancy in communication equipment to include land lines, cellular phones, computers and 800 megahertz radios.[8] Hospitals have also successfully used Web sites to list patients currently under hospital care in an effort to provide a resource to families attempting to locate loved ones after a disaster (a Joint Commission requirement). The importance of this step was underscored by the experience of St. Vincent's Hospital in New York City, which was inundated with nearly 25,000 family and friends on September 11, 2001.

In prior disaster situations, effectively communicating with the media and utilizing various media communications has been extremely important. As an example, during Katrina, with the large number of evacuees to other cities and states, the newspaper was used to help communicate with employees. The Brinker Corporation and other firms ran ads in the *Dallas Morning News* to communicate with their Gulf Coast employees who had evacuated to the Dallas area.

Although it is time consuming to communicate with the media and provide updates on the disaster situation, it is necessary. It is important to identify a public relations or media expert to provide these updates and he or she should be part of the ERT. Positively communicating with the media and providing updates will often provide the details that show progress, which helps to calm the public. As an example, during times of large electrical outages, the power companies will report every few hours the number of businesses and homes out of service for the hour and the progress since the last report. With the outage number oftentimes reduced by the hour, the public sees the progress and knows the power companies are working to improve the situation. A few of the tried and true steps to effectively communicating with the media are listed below:

1. Include a public affairs or media expert on the ERT. Have one or two official spokespeople for the healthcare organization. Let everyone know who these official contacts are and all requests for media updates should be provided only by them.
2. The official spokesperson will respond to media requests. Reporters do not go away. Deal with the situation in an honest and straightforward manner.
3. Prepare in advance facts that can be quoted and will serve as the anchor and focus of the discussion with the media.
4. Maintain a media list with contact names and numbers so you know with whom you are speaking.
5. Focus on thoughtful positive responses, and explain how you are moving ahead and correcting the disaster situation at hand.

STEP 5: ORGANIZATIONAL RESUMPTION PLANNING

The next step is for the organization to resume offering services as soon as possible even if they may be offered in a different location or on a smaller scale. The organizational resumption plan (ORP) focuses on how to recreate and maintain essential processes. The ORP provides procedures for recovering operations during or immediately following a disaster. These processes may possibly be at a remote location and at a time when normal operations and processes are not available. The organizational resumption plan will include many of the detailed responses to the questions that follow:

1. Under what situations and by whose authority will the business relocate to another location?
2. Is there another organization that can provide reciprocity of assistance such as facilities, equipment, personnel, communications capabilities or supplies?
3. What are the vendors, partners or secondary locations to consider when the primary location is no longer available?
4. Under what situation and by whose authority will the organization relocate back to the primary location?
5. What scheduling must be completed before moving back to the primary location?
   - Building renovation
   - Utilities
   - Employee moves
   - Testing of facilities and systems
   - Equipment relocation and set-up

STEP 6: TESTING AND AUDITING

Although the plan may be well constructed and documented on paper, it is important to test the plan with either a simulated or real-life situation. As a general rule, all continuity plans should be tested annually and more frequently if there are changes in the services, systems, employees, processes and procedures. Testing of the plan can be accomplished in a variety of methods. One process that could be used is known as a *table top exercise*[16] in which individuals discuss a hypothetical disaster and the necessary disaster recovery process and procedures. On the other extreme, hot site testing can occur when systems are actually taken off line, primary electrical sources are turned off and back-up electricity sources are brought on line in an attempt to create the issues that will occur during the disaster situation. Other testing methods that can be used are warm and cold site testing, which include more testing steps than the table top and fewer testing details than the hot site testing discussed. In the healthcare sector testing and auditing must include drills in addition to planning and training. The types of disasters are varied and include weather events, weapons of mass destruction or "dirty" bombs, bioterrorism, chemical spills or pandemics. It is impossible to train for all contingencies, and part of the strategic imperative is to drill for events more likely to happen. The Joint Commission requires hospitals to test emergency preparedness plans twice a year and one of the tests must be a part of a community-wide drill.[8]

STEP 7: PLAN MAINTENANCE

The final step—plan maintenance—is as important as creating the plan. Maintaining a plan with current and accurate information on assets, employee contacts, vendor contacts, up-to-date insurance plan information and coverage, test results and enhancements is mission critical. Although it is easy to simply say "yes, we have a plan" and check it off the list, a grossly outdated plan is like having no plan. On completion of the seven planning steps, the organization can review the Readiness Index score to identify future work to improve continuity and disaster preparedness.

SUMMARY

History has taught us that healthcare organizations and the communities in which they operate face a wide variety of potential disasters. It is not possible for healthcare organizations to prepare for all contingencies, and therefore they should take a strategic approach in allocating resources. This seven-step straight-forward approach to continuity and disaster recovery planning makes it possible for healthcare organizations to determine their organizational readiness, prioritize and create a plan that improves the organization effectiveness in times of disaster. The organization that is prepared and ready for a disaster is better positioned to provide critical support to clients in need. Managers and analysts play a key role in developing and updating these plans on a continuous basis.

References

1. Feldstein P. *Health Policy Issues, Third Edition.* Chicago: Health Administration Press; 2003.
2. PricewaterhouseCoopers' Health Research Institute. *Closing the Seams: Developing an Integrated Approach to Health System Disaster Preparedness.* 2007. Available at: www.pwc.com. Accessed online April 14, 2008.
3. Meyer-Emerick N, Momen M. Continuity planning for nonprofits. *Nonprofit Management and Leadership.* 2003; 14(1):67-77.
4. Wells A, Walker C, Walker T. *Disaster Recovery Principles and Practices.* Upper Saddle River, NJ: Prentice Hall; 2007.
5. Harris S. *All-in-One CISSP Exam Guide.* New York: McGraw-Hill/Osborne; 2008.
6. U.S. Department of Health and Human Services, Agency for Healthcare Research and Quality. *Reopening Shuttered Hospitals to Expand Surge Capacity.* Washington, DC; 2006.
7. U.S. Department of Homeland Security. *Pandemic Influenza: Preparedness, Response, and Recovery.* Washington, DC; September 19, 2006.
8. Meyers S. Disaster preparedness: Hospitals confront the challenge. *Trustee.* 2006; 59(2):12-19.
9. Thompson N, Gorder C. Health executives' role in preparing for the pandemic influenza 'gap': A new paradigm for disaster planning? *Journal of Healthcare Management.* 2007; 52(2):87-93.
10. Sather J, DiNiccola. Ready for trouble. *Health Facilities Management.* 2007; 20(2):23-28.
11. Romano M. At capacity and beyond. *Modern Healthcare.* 2005; 35(39):6-8.
12. Becker C. Five years later. *Modern Healthcare.* 2006; 36(36):10.
13. Blanke S, McGrady E. How to keep going when the going gets tough; Nonprofit Continuity planning in preparation for organizational disruption. *Conference Proceedings of the International Academy of Business and Public Administration Discipline.* 2007; 4(2), 306-316.
14. Blanke S, McGrady E. Are Not-for-Profit Organizations Ready for the Next Big Disaster? The 7 Steps to Straight-forward Business Continuity Planning for Not-for-Profit Organizational Readiness. *Southwest Decision Support Institute 2008 Annual Conference.* 2008.
15. Whitman M, Mattord H. *Principles of Incident Response and Disaster Recovery.* Boston: Thomson Course Technology; 2007.
16. Nemzow M. Business continuity planning. *International Journal of Network Management.* 1997; 7:127-136.
17. Harris S. *All-in-One CISSP Exam Guide.* New York: McGraw-Hill/Osborne; 2005.

CHAPTER 12

Service Level Agreements: Tools for Negotiating and Sustaining IT Performance

Guy Scalzi and Roger Kropf

> *"The purpose of business is to create and keep a customer."*
> — Peter Drucker, Professor of Management

INTRODUCTION

Some organizations have developed a written contract called a *service level agreement* (SLA) with an external vendor or an internal department. These agreements quantify what users can expect and allow the provider to be held accountable. We define SLAs and how they can be negotiated and used to measure and manage performance, as well as how to create a feedback loop to improve performance. We consider the potential positive and negative effects of SLAs, how specific dimensions of service can be measured and the costs that are involved. Our focus is information technology, but SLAs can be used to manage a variety of internal services performed in organizations, such as internal and external contracting for building maintenance, cycle time and costs for medical supplies in supply chains, and project expectations from performance improvement teams with user departments in key projects.

WHAT IS AN SLA?

Service Level Agreements define standards of performance for essential IT services. The term *service level agreement* is commonly used to describe the indicators, objectives or targets that are included in the service level agreement itself. Table 12-1 shows two examples of SLA metrics, one related to the performance of an electronic medical record (EMR) and one for a supply chain inventory system.

Service level agreements establish performance criteria on the front end of a relationship so there are no surprises as the relationship progresses. The SLA contract will stipulate a means to measure and report status and progress. Service level agreements often include a mechanism for addressing and improving poor performance, including

Table12-1: Sample Service Level Metric

Service	Service Level	Service Metric	Metric %
Electronic medical record	Screen refresh	Sub-second	100%
Supply chain inventory system	Inventory availability	Fulfillment rate	>98%

financial penalties. Service level agreements are the mechanism, or scorecard for monitoring ongoing performance and driving a continuous improvement environment. They can vary on the basis of type of service and can drive pricing or costs. Higher service levels command higher prices. Using objective measurement of IT services helps "substitute reality for subjective perception."[1]

DECISIONS

Decisions about SLAs need to be made only after answering the following important questions:

Should we be using SLAs? With just external vendors or internally? Service level agreements are important for setting expectations and replacing attitudes and anecdotes with empirical data. Using the excuse "IT never delivers" or "I don't have what I need to get my work done" is no longer acceptable when SLAs quantify what users can expect and allow the IT provider to be held accountable. Accountability and performance are as important for an internal IT department as they are for an outsourced provider. Using SLAs internally provides benefits including increased user satisfaction and productivity, increased consumer satisfaction, and an increase in IT staff productivity.[2] Service level agreements are important for an outsourced provider because these agreements compel their customers to define their expectations.

To appropriately set expectations, it is important to make clear who the customers and the providers are. For example, IT may enter into an agreement with the finance department, but delivery of the service actually depends on an external vendor. The finance department should understand that and recognize that IT's role is to manage the vendor relationship and that the IT department itself cannot guarantee delivery of the service. The ultimate provider may be an external vendor even when the agreement is between IT and the finance department.

Can managers and users really define SLAs? Aren't they technical—about the performance of the hardware and software? Who should write them? Service level metrics that are important to departments or business units, such as the availability of applications vital to work, should be included in formal agreements. Department or business unit staff should be involved in writing SLAs so it is more likely that their expectations are met and they begin to understand the cost of providing the level of service they want. Service level agreements about the performance of hardware and software should be included when they are directly related to getting users the services they want.

Are there other reasons to write SLAs besides saving money? There are other compelling reasons to write SLAs. They include regulatory compliance, patient safety, quality and the need to meet or exceed the performance of competitors.

What level of management needs to be involved? The manager one level up from the unit whose performance is affected needs to be involved. An SLA about the payroll system will be monitored by the payroll manager, but the finance director also needs to be involved. They need to know what the SLAs are, monitor them and be involved in decisions about performance improvement. This helps ensure that the process is taken seriously.

MAJOR ELEMENTS

Service level agreements should include four key elements including:
1. **Purpose:** What is the overall purpose of the measure (what is it trying to impact)?
2. **Description of service/duration:** SLAs should articulate clearly what the service level is and how long it will be measured.
3. **Metrics:** SLAs should include defined metrics (the exact goals or expectations).
4. **Payment and termination:** SLAs should articulate payment terms (if applicable) and outline conditions for termination if performance measures are missed.

CHARACTERISTICS

Department or business unit staff and the service provider must understand the SLA. Simpler and more focused SLAs are desirable. Vague or misleading SLAs serve no one, whereas clarity brings value to all parties. The measurement should be applicable. It should apply to what is being measured, correlate well with the customer's perception and be something the service provider will change. Service level agreements create value only when they accurately represent service delivery in a given environment. This is not simple to accomplish. A measure such as "low packet loss" is precise but may not be understood by managers outside of IT. Availability and even latency is easier to understand, but neither measure reflects the same dimension of quality.

The timeline for measurement should be coordinated with department or business unit expectations. Performance should not be measured selectively, and measurement should be automated wherever possible. Aggregation should not be used to hide problems. Further, SLAs should not be selected because the data are easily collected, but because they are useful (for example, to identify and remedy process problems).

The department or business unit and the service provider need to reach agreement on what will be measured and how. If the SLA involves availability, the period of time which is involved (a week, a month) should be stated. Will scheduled maintenance be excluded or included in calculating "uptime" for an application? (For the department or business unit, loss of an application for any reason is "downtime," even when it is scheduled).[3]

Be careful about insisting on SLAs that use measures that are different from the ones used internally by the service provider. Take a look at what the service provider uses to measure quality, because they are more likely to measure those well. If the measures are acceptable, do not require different ones that the service provider may measure poorly or at greater cost. Remember that they are training staff and maintaining systems to create their internal measures.[3]

The objective set in the SLA should be affordable (i.e., possible at a cost acceptable to the client).[2] While a client might desire that a system be available 99.999999% of the time, that level might not be possible at a cost the client is willing to pay, whereas 99.9% meets that test.

The SLA must represent something that is controllable. The "service provider must have the ability to exercise control over the factors that determine the level of service delivered."[2] Exclusions or waivers should be considered for factors that cannot be controlled. If the telephone company fails to honor a commitment to install phone lines to a building, the provider of IT services cannot be held accountable.

Both parties must agree to the SLA: for example, 80% of total help desk calls will be answered by a live agent within 30 seconds. The client must understand the service, metric and measurement, and the understanding of the services provided should match the customer's expectations. Unrealistic or unreasonable expectations damage the client/ provider relationship. While it may appear attractive for the customer to ask that 100% of total calls should be answered within 60 seconds, just one failure would mean that the provider had "failed" for that period. This may be an unreasonable expectation for IT but also offers no incentive for staff to comply for the rest of the reporting period.

NEGOTIATING SLAs

Establishing SLAs between two parties is always challenging. Barriers exist that must be worked through in order to form a successful relationship. Current performance must be evaluated to establish new service levels, and this is often difficult to measure because of a lack of data. In addition, negotiating and defining SLAs is challenging because processes and tools often do not exist to enable measurement. These must be worked through and understood by both parties. SLAs can be difficult to measure and organizational and process issues can sometimes impede an organization's ability to effectively measure. These process issues must also be addressed when establishing reasonable SLAs.

Three major considerations must be kept in mind during the negotiation:[1]

- **The benefits of a desired service level.** It is necessary for the user of the service to understand the impact of a given service level and keep in mind the limits of the cost and performance trade-off parameters.
- **The cost of delivering a given service level.** It is also necessary for the provider of the service to have a good understanding of the cost consequences of providing a specific level of service and to be able to justify the cost increase during the negotiation.
- **The availability of metrics.** The provider of the service must be aware of its capabilities to accurately measure the service level using metrics. If, as is often the case, satisfactory data cannot be collected, the service provider must be prepared to explain what should be done and what cost will be incurred by adding a data collector.

If SLAs are used internally, then agreements should be reached one client at a time. "This ensures that the IT manager, acting in the role of service provider to various lines of business, can furnish the maximum attention to each client. It also guards against the confusion—and ultimately, the political upheaval and rebellion—that can erupt when multiple departments clamor at once to grasp new technology."[2]

EFFECT ON BEHAVIOR

Service level agreements, if implemented correctly, can impact organizational behavior.[5,6] For instance, they bring direct accountability by measuring performance and identifying areas for improvement. They help clients by setting clear expectations and also presenting them with a reliable standard of service. The department or business unit can use SLAs to separate perception from reality when it comes to evaluating services performed. And finally, SLAs allow the IT department to "sell" a certain level of service to its clients with confidence and be assured (within reason) of continuous improvement.

Too much of a focus on SLAs can cause resources to be concentrated on minimizing the negative in specific areas while ignoring improvement in others. A focus on quickly resolving user problems can take the place of efforts to educate department or business unit staff, for example.

MEASURING SLAs: ESTABLISHING A BASELINE

One of the most important components in developing an appropriate SLA is to understand current performance before establishing future measurement guidelines. If this is not analyzed, the target performance measures that are established might not be attainable. In addition, clarifying objectives and communicating them broadly is critical.

Service level agreements should not be a distraction. Only that which is meaningful should be measured so that administrative costs are reduced. There should be fewer SLAs with higher rewards or penalties.

MEASUREMENT TOOLS

There should be a defined strategy for capturing data and creating reports. Having the right tools in place to measure service levels is critical. When possible, automated tools should be used to measure automated processes. Tools do exist in many areas including network performance, platform availability and critical server uptime. For example, the "uptime" of critical servers can be measured by using server logs and continuous "ping" tests. In this case, ping implies "Packet INternet Groper," which is "an Internet utility used to determine whether a particular IP (Internet protocol) address is reachable online by sending out a packet and waiting for a response. Ping is used to test and debug a network as well as see if a user or server is online."[4]

For non-automated processes, people close to the situation (those who actually perform the processes) should be employed to measure them. These people will be the best educated on the SLAs, the processes being measured and their importance to their organization.

COST OF SLAs

Sturm, Morris and Jander[2] identified the primary costs associated with implementing service level agreements. These include:

- IT personnel to plan, implement, monitor and report against service level agreements
- Software costs for purchasing or developing tools to monitor, diagnose, manage and report service quality, including problem notification
- Hardware costs for additional servers, workstations and specialist equipment for supporting the service management software tools
- IT management attention to justify, procure software and hardware, recruit and educate staff and oversee the operation of a service level management function

When SLAs are used in an outsourcing contract, the costs may not be visible to the client but still exist and are included in the cost of the agreement. However, large outsourcing organizations may incur lower costs because of existing licensing arrangements and the experience of their staff with these tools.

Software and hardware costs related to service level management will differ greatly according to the scale of the organization. A centralized IT organization that services multiple facilities will need more expensive tools than a single hospital. Software monitoring tools may be included in the purchase price of some hardware (for example, network routers). Organizations may need to acquire software reporting tools to merge and organize the data produced by existing hardware and software.

Real-time data are needed by service providers to avoid paying penalties. If an SLA requires that the provider meet a target each month, current status is needed to allow time for corrective action.

SUMMARY

Service level agreements can be used to measure services performed both internally and externally. In healthcare, the use of SLAs should be significantly expanded for a variety of functions and efforts, such as establishing agreed-on metrics and standards for achieving success in a specific project. In this chapter, we have concentrated on how service level agreements should be used for IT, which for management engineering professionals is one of the largest opportunities for process redesign. A sample SLA is shown in Figure 12-1, with a variety of metrics for use across all segments of IT. Developing and measuring SLAs such as these are essential to improving performance in health systems.

RESOURCES

Professionals interested in finding other resources on service level agreements should also explore the following Web sites:

- ITIL is the acronym for the "IT Infrastructure Library" guidelines developed by the Office of Governance Commerce (OGC) in Norwich, England, for the British government. It is considered by some the principal standard for service management. (www.itil.org/en/)
- Links to SLM software compiled by Bitpipe, Inc. (http://www.bitpipe.com/olist/Service-Level-Management.html)
- An example of the use of SLAs by the University of Michigan Plant Operations, which has an SLA in place with the University of Michigan Hospital for

Service	Item	Individual SLA	Metric %	Service Metric
Support Center/ Help Desk	1	Help desk first call resolution	65.00%	Resolution of calls at first contact, that are within scope
	2	Answer time	80.00%	Answered w/in 30 seconds
	3	Abandoned call	<5%	Max. calls abandoned over 20 secs.
	4	User satisfaction survey	80.00%	Minimum monthly avg. survey score
Data Center Services	5	Data backup	99.00%	Backups completed w/in schedule time
	6	Data restore	100%	Successful restores completed within time
	7	Server availability	Mission critical at 99.5%	Total measure of availability for mission and non-mission critical servers
	8	Disaster recovery testing	100%	Scheduled activities and testing completion
Network Services	9	Network performance	99.00%	Network backbone availability
	10	Equipment/Software release management	99.00%	Installs completed as scheduled
Desktop Services	11	Break/fix resolution	98.00%	Successful resolution within 1 business day
	12	Moves/adds/changed	99.00%	Successful completion within 10 business days

Figure 12-1: Sample IT SLA Standards and Metrics

maintenance/engineering support and a cyclical painting program. (http://www.plantops.umich.edu/PlantExchange/2003-winter/11.html)

- Nextslm.org is a Web site on SLM sponsored by BMC Software. (www.nextslm.org)
- A Web site on SLM is sponsored by Enterprise Management Associates. (http://www.emausa.com and select SLM from the technology areas listed)
- The IT Services Service Level Agreement (including individual SLAs) developed by Information Technology Services at the University of Washington School of Medicine. (http://home.mcis.washington.edu/amcis/services)
- A template used in writing an SLA for data center services by Information Technology Services at the Stanford University School of Medicine is available online. This is the template for a contract, but it includes SLAs. (http://med.stanford.edu/irt/datacenter/sla.html)

References

1. Garbani JP. *Best Practices for Service-Level Management.* Cambridge, MA: Forrester; 2004.
2. Sturm R, Morris W, Jander M. *Foundations of Service Level Management.* Indianapolis, IN: Sams; 2000.
3. Ferniany W. CEO University Hospitals and Clinics, The University of Mississippi Medical Center. Personal communication; 2007.
4. TechWeb.com. Definition obtained via TechEncyclopedia online at www.techweb.com; 2008.
5. Kropf R, Scalzi G. *Making Information Technology Work: Maximizing the Benefits for Healthcare Organizations.* Chicago: Health Forum/AHA Press; 2007.
6. Runyon B. *Service-Level Management for Care Delivery Organizations.* Stamford, CT: Gartner. March 30, 2007. ID Number: G00147472.

Glossary of Key Terms

Arrival event
A term used in queuing theory to describe when an entity arrives to the system.

As-is process
Process map that depicts the actual, current process in place prior to any process engineering.

Average length of stay
The average number of days a patient stays, from admission to discharge. An inpatient metric, which is calculated as the number of patient days during a period divided by the number of discharges. Also known as ALOS.

Benchmarking
Comparison of a key performance measurement relative to the competition or other leading organizations. The process of seeking best practices among better performing organizations, with intentions of applying those internally.

Benefit
Those gains in performance accrued to a process as a result of focused effort from a well-coordinated project. Perceived value that will be achieved with new service or technology.

Benefit realization
The process and guidelines for measuring and assuring that a project or program delivers expected performance benefits (e.g., stated goals).

Bottleneck
A choke point, or the point in a process at which capacity is limited, and which effectively reduces the number of outputs due to physical or logical constraints.

Capacity
The amount of resources or assets that exist to serve the demand.

Change
Transition from one state to another state, or a process of becoming different.

Coefficient of variation
A measure of variability, defined as the standard deviation divided by the mean.

Confidence interval
A term used in statistics and in simulation modeling. Provides a confidence estimate (i.e., $100 - \alpha\%$) where the mean of a process falls within the interval.

Continuity planning
Methods and procedures for dealing with longer-term outages and disasters. Includes performing business in a different mode and dealing with customers, partners and stakeholders through different channels until regular conditions are back in place.

De-bottleneck
To eliminate constraints or obstacles that limit capacity or throughput.

Defect
An instance in which a process fails to meet the customer's requirement.

Defect per million opportunities
A Six Sigma term defined as the # (number) of defects in a process divided by the total number of opportunities for defects, multiplied by 10^6. This term is used to convert to a Six Sigma Level (e.g., 1, 2, 3, etc) at which 3.4 DPMO is 6 Sigma and 691,500 DPMO is 1 Sigma. Also known as DPMO.

Disaster
Any occurrence that has a detrimental effect on an organization and disrupts the organization's ability to function.

Disaster recovery
Minimizing the effects of a disaster by taking necessary steps beforehand to ensure that resources can resume normal operations in a timely manner.

Discovery
A thorough investigation of the present environment and collection of evidence.

Evidence
Empirical data, or proof, supporting a decision or position.

Evidence-based healthcare
A philosophy that providing quality care is based on the current best scientific evidence, clinical judgment, and patient preference. Also known as EBHC.

Electronic health information system
A clinical system that includes aspects, such as order entry, patient records, reporting systems, access to information and decision support tools. Also known as EHIS.

General distribution
A term used in queuing theory. Describes an unknown distribution that requires estimation of the mean and standard deviation.

Goals
Broad, long-term statements of an ideal future state. The improvement amount the organization is trying to achieve.

Improve
To make something better. Positive change.

Kendall's notation
A term used in queuing. Notation scheme that displays information to describe the queue, such as distribution types, number of services and capacity (e.g., M/M/1).

Key performance indicators
A limited number of performance metrics that quantify operating results in critical areas, typically focused around strategic outcomes or productivity.

Lean
Process focused on quality improvements that increase speed, improve flexibility, reduce lot sizes, increase customization and reduce waste.

Low hanging fruit
Benefits that will be easily captured by focusing on those process steps that are the least costly and complex to rapidly improve.

Management engineering
A discipline focused on designing optimal management and information systems and processes, using tools from engineering, mathematics and social sciences. Application of engineering principles to healthcare processes. Also known as ME.

Metric
Measurement that includes a distinct numerator and denominator developed specifically to measure the established goal or objective.

Mission accountability
Holding non-profit organizations directly accountable for achieving their missions. A component of organizational performance in healthcare that aligns community and organization goals.

Morbidity
A measure of the rate of illness.

Mortality
A measure of the rate of incidence for deaths.

Objectives
Specific, short-term, quantifiable statements that are readily measurable.

Operational excellence
A term used to describe an organization that continuously seeks to improve its productivity, business processes and overall effectiveness.

Performance
The attainment of key goals, strategic advantage, or other outcomes desirable to an organization. Measured by outcomes, such as financial margins, quality, and satisfaction.

Performance improvement
A process or function devoted to creating positive change in outcomes, or transitioning from a steady state to something better. A methodology for adding value and delivering benefits in specific performance areas.

Portfolio management
A term used with regards to project management. The systematic governance of projects with an aim toward maximizing value or utility across the organization, while managing risks.

Process
A set of activities and tasks that are performed in sequence to achieve a specific outcome.

Process capability index
A measure for gauging the extent to which a process meets the customer's expectations (typically expressed as C_p or C_{pk}).

Process engineering
The careful scrutiny of a current state process to identify value creation opportunities, such as eliminating hand-offs or steps in the process.

Process flowchart
Diagram depicting the flows or activities in a process.

Productivity
The ratio of outputs to inputs for a specific process or system.

Project
An organized effort involving a sequence of activities that are temporarily being performed to achieve a desired outcome.

Project management
The application of knowledge, skills, tools and techniques to a project to achieve project success.

Project management office
A group of professionals that assists management in developing structure and standards for more sophisticated management of projects, especially those in information technology.

Project manager
The individual who leads the planning and daily activities necessary to achieve the project deliverables.

Prototype
A systems development approach that emphasizes rapid application design, in which users and developers work collaboratively to shorten development lead times.

Queuing theory
The science of waiting in line. The understanding of behaviors of wait times.

Relative value unit
Weighted volume unit typically used in ancillary and other departments in which traditional volume counts vary dramatically in terms of length, complexity or intensity of service provided.

Return on investment

A measure of the total project return that expresses the relationship between benefits and costs, which is expressed in discounted dollar values over time. Also known as ROI.

Risk

The uncertainty of events or outcomes. Possibility of suffering harm or loss, as during disasters.

Risk analysis

The process of analyzing threats and vulnerabilities.

Root cause analysis

Process for identifying and correcting the major issues causing problems.

Scorecard

A tool used by an organization to visualize measurements of key performance indicators relative to time, targets or other baselines. Also referred to as 'dashboards.'

Simulation

A logical or mathematical model of complex systems. A computer-based modeling technique used as an abstract representation of a real system.

Six Sigma

Methodology focused on improving processes and quality by eliminating defects and reducing variability or volatility of outcomes.

Stationary

A term used in queuing to indicate that the process mean does not change over time.

Surge capacity

The ability to rapidly expand services to meet increased demand, especially during times of disaster.

Target

A performance value that an organization is trying to achieve through a plan or project.

Throughput

The rate or velocity at which services are performed, or goods are delivered. Refers to the amount of outputs that a process can deliver over a specific time period and is used in both productivity analysis and process engineering.

Time and motion study

Analysis of the details of a process to identify the total amount of time and effort required to perform a procedure.

To-be process

A version of a process map that depicts the future state, or the state that will be achieved after design and process engineering.

Validation
The term used in modeling to describe the act of ensuring that the model reflects reality.

Variability
Inconsistency or dispersion of results. Variability in process outcomes is the major source of operational inefficiency and should be minimized as much as possible. Measured by standard deviation, or coefficient of variation.

Wait time
Time interval during which there is a temporary cessation of service.

Acronyms Used in This Book

ADE	adverse drug event
AHIC	American Health Information Community
ALOS	average length of stay
AOB	adjusted occupied bed
CAD	computer-aided design
CCHIT	Certification Commission for Healthcare Information Technology
CFO	chief financial officer
CIO	chief information officer
CMS	Centers for Medicare & Medicaid Services
CP	continuous planning
CPM	critical path method
CPOE	computerized practitioner order entry
CSO	customer service representative
DES	discrete-event simulation
DICE	duration, integrity, commitment, effort
DMAIC	define, measure, analyze, improve, control (Six Sigma)
DPMO	defect per million opportunities
EBHC	evidence-based healthcare system
ED	emergency department
EHIS	electronic health information system
EHR	electronic health record
EMR	electronic medical record
ERI	emergency response individual
ERP	emergency response plan
ERP	enterprise resource planning
FPA	finance, productivity, strategic alignment framework
FTE	full-time equivalent
GDP	gross domestic product
HASP	Healthcare Alliance Safety Partnership
HHS	U.S. Department of Health & Human Services
HR	human resources
IA	impact analysis
ICU	intensive care unit
IOM	Institutes of Medicine

IP	Internet protocol
IT	information technology
KPI	key performance indicator
LOS	length of stay
MAST	Multidisciplinary Antimicrobial Stewardship Team
ME	management engineer or management engineering
MRN	medical record number
NPV	net present value
ONC	Office of the National Coordinator of Health Information Technology
OR	operating room
ORP	organizational resumption plan
PACS	picture archiving and communications systems
PDCA	Plan-Do-Check-Act
PERT	program evaluation and review techniques
PI	performance improvement
PMO	project management office
PTO	personal time off
RFP	request for proposal
ROI	return on investment
RVU	relative value unit
SBC	stationary backlog carryover
SLA	service level agreement
SOA	service-oriented architecture
VNA	Visiting Nurses Association
WBS	work breakdown structure

Appendix:
Productivity Outputs Typical
Units of Measure for Healthcare*

Cost Center	Output (Workload Unit)
Nursing Administration	
Nursing—administration	Patient days, calendar days, # employees
Nursing—in-service education	# Employees, # new employees
Float nursing personnel	# Open positions, # unfilled shifts
Central transport	# Trips made
Nurses' Stations – Medical and Surgical Acute	
Designated medical and surgical acute care units	Patient days, modified by acuity
Pediatric acute	Patient days, modified by acuity
Psychiatric acute	Patient days, modified by acuity
Other adult and pediatric acute detoxification unit(s)	Patient days, modified by acuity
Communicable disease unit(s)	Patient days, modified by acuity
Obstetric (gynecological) acute	Patient days, modified by acuity
Newborn nursery acute premature unit(s)	Patient days, modified by acuity
Intensive care	Patient days, modified by acuity
Medical-surgical intensive care unit(s)	Patient days, modified by acuity
Pediatric intensive care unit(s)	Patient days, modified by acuity
Neonatal intensive care unit(s)	Patient days, modified by acuity
Definitive observation intensive care unit(s)	Patient days, modified by acuity
Psychiatric (isolation) intensive care unit(s)	Patient days, modified by acuity
Burn care	Patient days, modified by acuity
Cardiac Care	
Myocardial infarction unit(s)	Patient days, modified by acuity
Pulmonary care unit(s)	Patient days, modified by acuity
Heart transplant unit(s)	Patient days, modified by acuity

* Adapted from Gray SP, Steffy W. *Hospital Cost Containment through Productivity Management*. New York: Van Nostrand Reinhold Co; 1983; 203-208.

Extended (long-term) and other care:	
Skilled nursing unit(s)	Patient days, modified by acuity
Rehabilitation unit(s)	Patient days, modified by acuity
Long-term psychiatric unit(s)	Patient days, modified by acuity
Residential unit(s)	Patient days, modified by acuity
Self-care unit(s)	Patient days, modified by acuity
Hemodialysis	# Treatments, # patients
Respiratory Services	
Respiratory therapy	# Treatments, # ventilator patients, # relative value units
Pulmonary function testing	# Tests
Labor and Delivery Services	
Labor room(s)	# Deliveries, # C-sections, # antepartum patients
Delivery room(s)	# Deliveries, # C-sections, # antepartum patients
Surgical services:	
General surgery	# Patients, # procedures, # OR minutes
Organ transplants	# Patients, # procedures, # OR minutes
Open-heart surgery	# Patients, # procedures, # OR minutes
Neurosurgery	# Patients, # procedures, # OR minutes
Orthopedic surgery	# Patients, # procedures, # OR minutes
Minor surgery	# Patients, # procedures, # OR minutes
Surgical day care	# Patients, # procedures, # OR minutes
Recovery room(s)	# Patients, # procedures
Emergency Services	
Emergency department	# Visits, # trauma visits
Ambulance service	# Trips
General Services	
Central services	Patient days, # OR procedures, line items cleaned
Central sterile supply	Patient days, # OR procedures, line items cleaned
Laboratory Services	
Chemistry	# Patients, # procedures, # relative value units
Hematology	# Patients, # procedures, # relative value units
Histology	# Patients, # procedures, # relative value units
Autopsy	# Patients, # procedures, # relative value units
Special procedures	# Patients, # procedures, # relative value units
Immunology	# Patients, # procedures, # relative value units
Microbiology	# Patients, # procedures, # relative value units

Radioisotopes	# Patients, # procedures, # relative value units
Procurement and dispatch	# Patients, # procedures, # relative value units
Urine and feces	# Patients, # procedures, # relative value units
Blood bank	# Patients, # procedures, # relative value units
Electrodiagnosis	
Electrocardiology	# Patients, # procedures, # relative value units
Electromyography	# Patients, # procedures, # relative value units
Electroencephalography	# Patients, # procedures, # relative value units
Imaging/Radiology – Diagnostic	
Angiocardiography	# Patients, # procedures, # relative value units
Imaging/Radiology – Therapeutic	
Chemotherapy	# Patients, # procedures, # relative value units
Radiation therapy	# Patients, # procedures, # relative value units
Nuclear Medicine	
Nuclear medicine – diagnostic	# Patients, # procedures, # relative value units
Nuclear medicine – therapeutic	# Patients, # procedures, # relative value units
Pharmacy	# Patients, # procedures, # relative value units
Anesthesiology	# OR patients, # OR minutes
Rehabilitation Services	
Physical therapy	# Treatment modalities, # visits, # relative value units
Occupational therapy	# Treatment modalities, # visits, # relative value units
Speech pathology (speech therapy)	# Treatment modalities, # visits, # relative value units
Recreational therapy	# Treatment modalities, # visits, # relative value units
Plant Operation and Maintenance Services	
Plant maintenance	Sq. feet maintained, # orders
Carpentry	Sq. feet maintained, # orders
Plumbing	Sq. feet maintained, # orders
Painting	Sq. feet maintained, # orders
Electrical and refrigeration operations	Sq. feet maintained, # orders
Automotive services	Sq. feet maintained, # orders
Plant operations	Sq. feet maintained, # orders
Grounds	Sq. feet maintained, # orders
Boiler and power plant	Sq. feet maintained, # orders
Parking	Sq. feet maintained, # orders
Elevator operation	Sq. feet maintained, # orders
Security	Sq. feet maintained, # orders

Housekeeping	Sq. feet maintained
Laundry and Linen Service	
Laundry service	Pounds processed
Linen service	Packs made
Admitting	# Admissions, # preadmissions, # transfers
Cashiering	# Visits, $$$
Credit and collections	# Accounts, $$$
Ambulatory Services	
Medical-surgical clinic	Outpatient visits
Eye, ear, nose, and throat clinic	Outpatient visits
Urology clinic	Outpatient visits
Obstetrics and gynecology clinic	Outpatient visits
Orthopedics clinic	Outpatient visits
Pediatric clinic	Outpatient visits
Surgery clinic	Outpatient visits
Cardiology clinic	Outpatient visits
Physical medicine clinic	Outpatient visits
Psychiatric clinic	Outpatient visits
Home Health Care	
Nursing service	Home care visits
Rehabilitation services	Home care visits
Social services	# Cases
Health information management/Medical records	Discharges, outpatient visits, emergency department visits
Medical library services	Linear feet maintained
Dietary Services	
Kitchen	# Meals
Dietitians/Patient food services	# Meals, # consultations
Cafeteria	# Meals
Administrative Services	
Management engineering	# Projects
Purchasing	# Purchase orders, $$$ purchases
Communications	# Calls, # pages
Printing and duplicating	# Copies made, # orders
Receiving and stores	# Deliveries
Human resources/Personnel	# Employees, # new employees
Employee medical services	# Employees, # new employees
Case management/Medical care evaluation	Discharges, outpatient visits, emergency room visits

Fiscal Services	
Fiscal services office	# Beds
General accounting	# Beds, # accounts
Budget and costing	# Beds
Payroll accounting	# Employees
Accounts payable	# Accounts
Plant and equipment	# Beds
Inventory accounting	# Beds
Patient accounting	# Discharges, # outpatient visits, # emergency department visits, # accounts
Information systems/Data processing	# Applications
Research	
Research administrative office	# Projects, $$$ funding
Hospital research projects	# Projects, $$$ funding
Joint research projects	# Projects, $$$ funding
Medical school research projects	# Projects, $$$ funding
Non-physician Education	
School of nursing – administrative offices	# Students
Registered nurse program	# Students
Licensed vocational (practical) nurse program	# Students
Medical Staff Service and Education	
Voluntary medical staff	# Staff members
Paid medical staff	# Staff members
Medical graduate education	# Staff members
General Measures	
Overall productivity	Adjusted admissions Adjusted discharges Adjusted patient days Adjusted occupied beds Salary expense per net revenue Supply expense per net revenue
Physician Office Measures	
Staff productivity	# Patient visits
Provider/staff productivity	# Weighted procedures
Insurance Division Measures	
Claims processing	# Claims processed per hour # Adjudicated claims # Rejected claims
Membership	Per member per month revenue Per member per month cost # New members # Renewal members

Index